# Clinician Technique in Personalized Psychotherapy

# Clinician Technique in Personalized Psychotherapy

by
**Mardi Horowitz, M.D.**

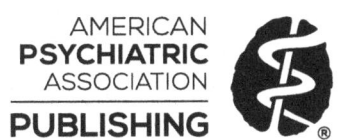

AMERICAN
**PSYCHIATRIC**
ASSOCIATION
**PUBLISHING**

Copyright © 2025 American Psychiatric Association Publishing
ALL RIGHTS RESERVED

First Edition

Manufactured in the United States of America on acid-free paper

29  28  27  26  25    5  4  3  2  1

American Psychiatric Association Publishing
800 Maine Avenue SW, Suite 900
Washington, DC 20024-2812
www.appi.org

**Library of Congress Cataloging-in-Publication Data**
Names: Horowitz, Mardi Jon, 1934- author.
Title: Clinician technique in personalized psychotherapy / Mardi Horowitz.
Description: First edition. | Washington, DC : American Psychiatric Association Publishing, [2025] | Includes bibliographical references and index.
Identifiers: LCCN 2025010670 (print) | LCCN 2025010671 (ebook) | ISBN 9798894551241 (paperback) | ISBN 9798894551258 (ebook)
Subjects: MESH: Psychotherapy--methods
Classification: LCC RC480.5 (print) | LCC RC480.5 (ebook) | NLM WM 420 | DDC 616.89/14--dc23/eng/20250430
LC record available at https://lccn.loc.gov/2025010670
LC ebook record available at https://lccn.loc.gov/2025010671

**British Library Cataloguing in Publication Data**
A CIP record is available from the British Library.

# Contents

# About the Author

**Mardi Horowitz, M.D., is Distinguished Professor of Psychiatry at the University of California San Francisco.**

## Disclosures

Mardi Horowitz, M.D., stated that he had no competing interests during the year preceding manuscript submission.

# Foreword

The path to becoming a good therapist is full of twists and turns and difficult passages. There are many talented therapists who do effective work with patients, but few can serve as excellent guides on this path—few can explain exactly what they do in therapy that works. This gap in teaching is often called the "art" of psychotherapy, as if it is a gift of intuition and creativity that talented therapists naturally develop, rather than a way of thinking and a set of skills that can be learned.

Fortunately, Mardi Horowitz has drawn on years of psychotherapy research and clinical practice to guide both new and experienced therapists on a clear and logical path through the complex course of treatment. Few therapists are able to explain the moment-to-moment choices we make, over the course of therapy, in a logical way. Nevertheless, those who read this book will likely recognize their own work in these pages and think: "This describes what I have been doing in my practice for years!"

*Clinician Technique in Personalized Psychotherapy* describes an integrative cognitive-psychodynamic approach that can be applied flexibly with patients from diverse backgrounds and with different diagnoses. This approach is an important guide for beginning therapists who are learning the foundational skills of supportive, cognitive-behavioral, and psychodynamic therapy. It is equally helpful for experienced therapists interested in learning an integrative approach to logically apply different interventions at different points in therapy. The book has been invaluable to me as I update my psychotherapy curriculum for child and adolescent psychiatry fellows, adding more clear explanations of how and when to use different interventions.

I have been fortunate to learn and practice psychotherapy, with both adults and children, at a time of explosive growth in options for treatment, including medications, other somatic treatments, and a wide range of psychotherapy approaches. When I began training in psychotherapy, my teachers shared a common psychodynamic perspective on how psychotherapy works, a theory that explained normal development and pathological development, and a treatment approach informed and guided by this theoretical model. The theory describes how our earliest relationships with caregivers shape our patterns of behavior, along with longings, frustrations, fantasies, and fears that persist into adulthood in unconscious form, hidden and inaccessible to conscious change. Change in these patterns of response occurs by making the unconscious conscious, as patient and therapist experience the emergence of these patterns in the present moment of the therapy relationship, in the form of transference. Transference makes the previously hidden source of these patterns accessible for recognition and revision by the patient, who is liberated from old longings and fears that exerted control from outside of awareness.

This psychodynamic approach, using free association and transference as gateways to the unconscious, offered a sense of clear direction and coherent guidance to its practitioners. Indeed, some patients experienced liberation from repetitive, maladaptive patterns. But the treatment was not compatible with the cognitive style, cultural experiences, or emotional needs of other patients who either experienced no change or became more troubled. For some patients, longings, fears, and impulses emerged and intensified in the transference, at times overwhelming the patient's (and the analyst's) ability to modulate the experience.

Adherence to this one approach could not address the suffering of the wide range of patients in need of treatment. As a young psychiatrist-in-training, I wondered why psychiatry was different from other medical and surgical practices, in which one expected to learn and apply a wide variety of interventions for different disorders, each of which could have different presentations depending on the condition of the individual patient and the timing of the progression or resolution of the illness. It seemed to make sense that, like our medical and surgical colleagues, all of us treating psychiatric disorders should have a variety of interventions to offer.

Fortunately, new understandings of the multiple, complex causes of emotional distress and new treatment approaches have evolved since we began to address suffering with talking therapy. These innovations have provided a wide range of treatment options for a diverse group of patients seeking treatment for a variety of disorders in the context of many different social, cultural, and economic settings. Because the typical practitioner does not have the opportunity to develop expertise in multiple highly specialized interventions, each psychotherapist has developed expertise in their favorite approach. In response, divisions have arisen among psychotherapists, with adherents of one approach competing—rather than collaborating—with others. Those who still long for a singular approach may argue that their approach is the best: it has the most randomized controlled trials, or addresses the root of the problem at its deepest source, or offers change in the most lasting way.

For the psychiatrist-in-training, the variety of treatment approaches can be overwhelming and discouraging. Why bother learning psychotherapy when there is not enough time to master multiple approaches? For educators and supervisors of psychotherapy, the proliferation of treatment styles has led to bewildering choices regarding how to teach the fundamentals of becoming a good psychotherapist. Should training programs offer students immersion in one approach, so that they can become skilled in addressing psychiatric problems in a particular way, with the option to learn other techniques after residency? Or should training programs offer a variety of approaches, with the risk that students will never develop expertise in any one form of therapy?

In contrast to this proliferation of too-many-techniques-to-learn, some innovative approaches are based on models that unify, rather than divide, the human experience. Among the approaches that have enriched our understanding and treatment of the causes of emotional suffering are the Unified Protocol for Transdiagnostic Treatment of Emotional Disorders (Barlow et al. 2017), Acceptance and Commitment Therapy (Hayes et al. 2011), and other mindfulness-based interventions. These approaches emphasize that change occurs through an experiential process, including exercises, access to feelings that cannot be expressed entirely in words, and learning and practicing new models of relationships to oneself, to others, and to the world.

What distinguishes the integrative process described in these pages from other unifying models is Horowitz's careful and detailed method for determining what techniques will be effective as the therapy progresses through different stages, through moment-to-moment collaboration between therapist and patient. As we learn this method of continual reassessment and response to the emerging process of therapy, we discover how to use well-researched, evidence-based interventions to deliver the personalized psychotherapy that each unique individual, and each unique therapist-patient dyad, will require. In addition, we recognize how to sustain a therapeutic approach with patients whose symptoms are not adequately addressed by somatic therapy or who may not be responding as hoped.

This book's integrative approach also helps establish common ground among faculty and psychotherapy supervisors who have different areas of expertise in cognitive-behavioral, behavioral, and psychodynamic therapy. Instead of offering competing approaches, instructors can collaborate on different approaches according to the needs of the patient and the supervisee at any point in treatment. Research based on observations of therapy sessions has confirmed what experienced therapists have learned: experts who specialize in a particular therapeutic approach routinely use techniques from other approaches (Ablon and Jones 1998). In the last two decades, psychotherapy outcome research has demonstrated positive outcomes with a variety of psychotherapy approaches, with no one specific technique contributing more to a good outcome than the positive therapeutic relationship (Duncan 2002; Norcross and Wampold 2018; Wampold 2015). If we are to take this body of research seriously, we should organize our teaching of therapy around our understanding of how the therapeutic alliance is maintained at each stage of treatment, as patient and therapist move collaboratively to their shared goals.

One of the most valuable lessons that I take from this book is a method for teaching how to strengthen the therapeutic alliance at any stage of treatment. Many clinicians will need to make recommendations for care based on brief assessments in the compressed time of an emergency room encounter or hospital consultation. Some will develop long-term therapeutic relationships over the course of medication-focused visits at infrequent intervals. Others will engage their patients in short- or long-term psychotherapy. All will benefit from the guidance in Table 1.1 in Chapter 1 ("Stages of Psychotherapy"), which describes the patient activities, therapist techniques, and methods for attending to the therapeutic relationship at each stage of treatment. Early in assessment, patient and family can develop a working relationship with the evaluator by agreeing on the goals and roles of each member in the collaborative relationship. Alliance-building is applicable across all psychiatric settings. As Table 1.2 suggests, "defin[ing] each party's roles in promoting safety while discussing negative emotional states" is an important starting point to stabilize symptoms in these settings.

The book excels at helping the reader reflect on many examples of challenging moments in therapy, with a wide range of patients at different stages of treatment. In the vivid case examples, Horowitz, like a helpful psychotherapy supervisor, offers suggestions while explaining how and why these choices can address the patient's needs at each stage of treatment. Each clinical example offers detailed explanations of how to respond and why one intervention might work better than another under the conditions of that moment in therapy. As a result, reading this book feels like meeting with a good supervisor who not only shares a set of guidelines that are understandable and doable but also generously offers examples of what statement, what tone of voice, and what facial expression will help modulate states of mind and repair ruptures in the therapeutic alliance at difficult moments. Here, in particular, experienced therapists will recognize those subtle adjustments of expression they have honed over the years through observing how their patients have responded to what they say and do.

Horowitz also normalizes the therapist's experience of responses that don't work as we intended, with guidance on how to deal with ruptures. The book describes how the therapist can use words and tone of voice to strengthen the therapeutic alliance and contain disruptive affective states for a patient struggling with sensitive issues. For me, the parallel processes of therapy and supervision came alive as I read. At the same time, I felt the containing and calming effect of having my struggles as a therapist validated and addressed by the rich clinical examples in the book.

In the book's preface and first two chapters, Horowitz explains the structure and process of psychotherapy. As a guide to conducting psychotherapy in a logical and patient-centered way, the model shows how the whole range of evidence-based treatments—including the teaching of skills, psychoeducation, cognitive-behavioral interventions, mentalizing, and psychodynamic understanding of transference—can be applied, as indicated, at different stages of treatment.

Several tables and diagrams helpfully organize the multitude of observations made in assessments or therapy sessions into manageable categories that guide interventions. It will be particularly beneficial for learners of psychotherapy to formally apply the configurational analysis, to diagram the evolving self-other schemas, and to assess positive states of mind and sense of self-regard. For those of us who don't always do things "by the book," it will still be of great benefit to reflect on these research-based—yet experience-near—approaches that guide assessment and intervention. For example, for much of my practice, I have been aware of the shifting states of mind in myself and my patients over the course of any therapy session. Yet I had not thought about how to use these observations intentionally, in a collaborative way, with patients experiencing different types of vulnerability. Nor had I figured out how to teach my supervisees a method of determining what type of intervention to use, across a wide variety of patients, based on a methodical assessment of where the patient is in the present moment.

Throughout every example of the therapist-patient interaction, we learn a style and attitude of respectful collaboration that can be used at every stage of treatment, with patients at all levels of self-reflection. Moments of potential rupture can become opportunities for strengthening the alliance and moving therapy forward with brief, thoughtfully worded reflections. These include simple reminders of respective roles in the collaborative process, the therapist's intentions and reasons for approaching difficult experiences, and instances in the therapy relationship when talking about dreaded topics has furthered the patient's goals.

We see how a patient's maladaptive patterns of relationships can be understood, explored, and changed as patient and therapist develop, deepen, and repair disruptions in their working relationship. We are given repeated examples of how to intentionally use the therapy relationship as both the supportive structure for doing difficult work and the essential mechanism for change. Through brief case narratives and simple diagrams, we see how a therapist's responses can help a patient recognize what has been maladaptive in their repetitive patterns in failed or destructive relationships. Through repeated experiences of being well supported in approaching feared emotions and topics in therapy, the patient learns to trust self and other in new relationship roles. The theme that shines through every example, growing more clear with each iteration, is how the therapist can enact and inspire respectful collaboration through words, behavior, and nonverbal expressions.

In Chapter 8 ("Confronting Dilemmas by Assertion of a Therapeutic Alliance"), Horowitz describes the all-too-familiar experience therapists feel when facing an "impossible" dilemma. I recall many examples in my own practice when a patient's pattern of response kept others at a distance when the patient was seeking closeness. I experienced the pattern being repeated in the therapy relationship with me, and I knew I needed to address it to help the patient recognize how they alienated others despite their conscious efforts to get closer. Yet I couldn't figure out how to raise the issue without offending the patient; I imagined that any mention of it would touch off a cascade of shameful feelings and rupture the relationship. In Chapter 8, Horowitz explains:

> Once a working state has been restored, a dilemma as experienced in the mind of the therapist can be shared with the patient. The therapist takes ownership of uncertainty (I statements) and does not place it on the patient (you statements).

He describes how the therapist can genuinely communicate: "I have a dilemma. I feel a bit unsure of what I should say to you." The therapist can explain both sides of the dilemma. While reading this example, I thought of how I could frame my dilemma with a patient whose longing for repeated reassurances of caring had become alienating to her family and friends, as well as overly demanding with me. I imagined how I might explain to the patient that I was aware that in observing my own limits (and not giving her the reassurance she felt she needed through frequent phone calls), I would leave her feeling neglected and ashamed of her request. Yet if I went along with her request, I would not be helping her with the pattern of behavior that was undermining her closest connections.

As a pathway from impossible dilemma to collaborative work, Horowitz suggests saying, "So I am unsure how to proceed; perhaps you are as well? I think we can clarify this together, slowly, piece by piece." This type of transparency and the invitation to rejoin the collaborative work of treatment could be helpful—not only with patients in individual therapy, but also with a younger patient's parents and family members, whose patterns of interaction can undermine the child's treatment if not addressed.

At times we are struck by the "just rightness" of a melody, a poem, or a work of art that seems so natural—so obvious—that it feels as if it has always been there, hidden in plain sight. Clinicians who use a variety of psychotherapy techniques in attuned response to patients may find that this book reveals a beautiful logic they have been unaware of using all along. While this discovery will be gratifying for the experienced clinician, it will be invaluable for the beginning therapist, who can begin practicing psychotherapy guided by the wisdom and clarity that is revealed to us by a skilled clinician.

Roberta Isberg, M.D.
Assistant Professor (Part Time) of Psychiatry, Harvard Medical School
Senior Attending Psychiatrist, Department of Psychiatry
and Behavioral Sciences, Boston Children's Hospital, Boston,
Massachusetts

# Preface

During psychotherapy, clinicians combine techniques from various modalities they learn from training, continuing education, and experience. This book aims to help them by considering how to understand the individual patient in the present. It serves as a guide for considering theory and practice as an integrative process of continuous formulation that individuals experience as they go through stages of psychotherapy.

My research involved decades of watching psychotherapy videotapes and figuring out what (if anything) changed and how, why, and when a person changed. This book is derived from my clinical practice, teaching, and supervising and provides essential ingredients and practical examples of what to say in therapy. Patients and therapists may stem from communities and families that are culturally different. As the patient and therapist converse, the hope is that they will come to share purposes and frameworks of belief. Confronting possibly different value systems can aid in building the most important aspect of change, the therapeutic alliance. Enriching the therapeutic alliance through deepening states of work with a patient is a topic across the chapters.

Consider the state of our field. The evidence-based therapies listed in treatment guidelines follow manuals that were used in the controlled research designs necessary to get funding for randomized clinical trials. These modalities were usually linked to a DSM diagnosis, and the treatments were usually time-limited to get the research done in a timely and fiscally efficient manner. In general, the effects of treatment were positive in symptom reduction but met only some goals in some patients. A clinician who does not need to adhere to the manual of a clinical trial has greater freedom to choose how to act and thus to tailor treatment to the patient's particular needs, strengths, and life circumstances.

This book is based on an integrative cognitive-psychodynamic theory about both conscious and unconscious meaning structures. Many patients might start with aims to ameliorate symptoms and social dysfunctions but advance in therapy to aims involving personality growth (Horowitz 2016a).

The book begins with a chapter on how a person may start therapy to address specific symptoms and complaints and proceed to explore the depths of emotional and relationship schemas. Chapter 1 ("Stages of Psychotherapy") addresses the reality of therapeutic technique—that it changes through stages as safety is increased. Therapy can be highly individualized by observing qualities of expression. Generally, it goes through stages. Deepening understanding, the therapist and patient together gradually modify the techniques the therapist uses. The chapter presents a model that begins with assessments and goes on to how to end the treatment.

Chapter 2 ("Formulating") and Chapter 3 ("Choosing What to Say in the Present Moment") provide ways for formulating and reformulating as stages of therapy progress. This approach is useful for clinicians who are trained in psychiatry, psychology, or counseling; they will recognize concepts from that training, which I have integrated by focusing on individualized formulations to personalize how to help a patient on the path of self-evolution.

A states-of-mind approach allows consideration of the motivations for safety and threat mastery even at the surface of conversations, before the depth of preconscious schemas is considered. In Chapters 1–3, a model of wish, fear, and defensive configurations provides the therapist with a frame for individualization, especially sharing a state-of-mind understanding with the patient.

Next, the schemas that organize states and maladaptive patterns in some states are considered. Chapter 4 ("Techniques When Obstacles Stall Progress") deals with techniques for understanding and ameliorating obstacles and defensive avoidances. Emotional blunting, intellectualization, generalization, and projections are discussed, with practical advice on how to ameliorate them without flooding or disorganization because of excessive emotional intensity and dysregulation. In Chapter 5 ("Paying Attention to the Patient's Current Level of Personality Functioning"), complex issues are addressed in terms of technical variation between patients who may have more dissociative experiences and those who can move well along a path of adaptive change. Techniques considered include showing adaptive routes forward and slowing down impulses.

Chapter 6 ("Correcting Schemas From Experiences in a Therapeutic Alliance") continues the topic of how to get at the beliefs within the schemas from a prior attachment and the theme of developing a safe frame of patient-therapist relationship, leading to adaptation in patients who have developed only an insecure pattern of attachment with others. Chapter 7 ("Managing Narcissistic Traits") addresses the difficult problems presented by patients with narcissistic traits. Handling anger in sessions, particularly when patients blame others, is important, as is helping the patient with their fear of shame states and incipient grief attacks. Learning from the new experiences in an enriched therapeutic alliance is again addressed as a technique of change to more secure models of relating to others. Chapter 8 ("Confronting Dilemmas by Assertion of a Therapeutic Alliance") describes how to deal with the dilemmas therapists commonly experience in deeper treatments. Once again, as in chapters integrating modalities of therapy by commonalities, the common current theoretical language of self and relationship schemas provides a general model (Diamond et al. 2022).

Assessing change is valuable as feedback to both patient and therapist. But it may also be valuable to look at improvements in states of mind. Chapter 9 ("Assessing Change During Treatment") provides ways to consider whether change is taking place in a language that emphasizes positive life experiences. The two simple self-report scales provided can be reproduced and used to track change, as supplements to the standard scales used for screening and tracking depression, anxiety, and PTSD by self-report. This chapter also describes techniques of termination in a way that sustains a sense of having had a therapeutic alliance.

The case examples throughout are fictionalized composites of multiple therapeutic encounters. On first use, key terms are in bold type and defined in footnotes; all the terms are listed in the Glossary of Terms, which precedes the Index.

# Acknowledgments

The research background for this book was supported by funding from three major sources:

- The University of California San Francisco (UCSF): I formed and directed the Psychotherapy Evaluation and Study Center in the Department of Psychiatry and Behavioral Sciences.
- The National Institute of Mental Health, National Institutes of Health: I formed and directed the Center for the Study of Neuroses in the UCSF Department of Psychiatry and Behavioral Sciences.
- The MacArthur Foundation: I formed and directed the Program on Conscious and Unconscious Mental Processes, an international collaboration centered in the UCSF Department of Psychiatry and Behavioral Sciences.

Zach Vanderbilt was extremely helpful in many aspects of this book, including insightful critiques, astute literature review, and editing. By editing the manuscript, Steven Walsh, M.D., supported clarity in exposition. I thank Renee Binder for all she has done for me personally and professionally.

Mardi Horowitz, M.D.
San Francisco, 2025

# Stages of Psychotherapy

Optimal processes in psychotherapy occur if a clinician uses techniques derived from an understanding of the current stage in treatment and formulates goals and actions according to the patient's characteristics. Personalization is achieved as each individual patient is modeled in the mind of the therapist as a whole person, in the context of their personal history and future aspirations.

The patient's expectations may be nuanced and layered and are likely to change as therapy progresses. The therapist's techniques are based on the evolution of the process of therapy and the patient's preferences. Generally, the stages of work go from the surface—listening to what patients say—to deeper levels—considering the patient's intentions and **preconscious**[1] plans for life.

Personalized formulating leads to the integration of techniques derived from various empirically studied modalities. The commonalities across types of therapy are chosen according to the understanding that develops about this patient's possibilities. Modifications of the work occur as treatment progresses. A typical evolution of therapy includes six stages:

- Assessment: A stage of psychotherapy in which complaints, signs, symptoms, problems in living, precipitants, perpetuations,

---

[1] Preconscious: Occurring before conscious representation.

protective resources, and predispositions are considered (and reconsidered).

- Support: A stage of therapy in which guidance, empathy, and psychoeducation are prominent.
- Exploration of meanings: A stage of therapy in which the significance of events to self and loved ones is expanded in terms of implications and expectations for the future.
- Re-narration: The process of going back over stories to register a revised, more realistic set of memories.
- Re-schematization: The process of altering belief structures by adding new elements, reorganizing existing elements, and altering linkage-strength patterns in the associational connection between elements. The result can modify personality-based attitudes and assumptions.
- Drawing to a close.

Some patients move quickly through the early stages of assessment and support. They explore meanings, express feelings related to ideas, and may re-narrate precipitants and perpetuators of their problems. They may not be motivated for further stages of therapy, which include re-schematization of **attachment models**[2] and **identity**.[3] The pace depends on the complexity of biopsychosocial factors, including the patient's current level of **personality**[4] functioning and their capacity to maintain a sense of safety while exploring difficult topics and feelings.

## Stages of Therapy

## Assessment

Assessment begins as the patient seeks present reasons for wanting treatment. Usually it is a stage of psychotherapy in which complaints,

---

[2] Attachment model: A preconscious schema of self as connected to significant others (such as parents) in development.

[3] Identity: Awareness of the self as a continuous, and usually coherent, entity that perceives, thinks, feels, decides, and acts. Conscious identity rests on belief structures of one's unconscious self-organization (see footnote 6).

[4] Personality: An individual's enduring and slowly changing configurations of beliefs, preferences, values, traits, and tendencies that make up a unique combination of potential moods, thoughts, and behaviors. Personality consists of the important components of identity and one's relationship patterns, as well as a person's capacity for emotional regulation.

signs, symptoms, and problems in living are considered. Assessment blends with supportive stages if a patient needs help coping with immediate circumstances and concerns such as housing and food. Subsequently, the therapist and patient can work together to explore meanings related to precipitating stressors. Later stages may address **repetitive maladaptive patterns**[5] and problems in **self-organization**[6] that are informed by preconscious coding, such as **schemas.**[7] This work usually expands to clarifying beliefs and feelings about self and relationships.

In assessment stages, the patient and clinician are learning about and from each other and attempting to develop a secure connection. Each of them may have some tentative hypotheses that are incomplete and not yet agreed on. A sequence of assessment, support, and exploration of meanings can lead to re-narration of past events and re-schematization of identity and attachment models. Together, the patient and therapist advance a **therapeutic alliance.**[8]

Some patients may express frustration about the therapeutic process, as in this example from the assessment stage:

*Therapist:* Let's talk about what you want to accomplish here.
*Patient:* I want to become a little happier [smiles wanly]. I lost a long-standing relationship. It didn't make me happy; I couldn't stand them. I'm lonely but get no pleasure from dinner with anyone.
*Therapist:* These topics of loss and your hopes to be happier in the future are possibly ones for us to explore further.
*Patient:* Where do I start? [silence]
*Therapist:* I thought I saw some tears in your eyes. What did you feel just then?

---

[5] Maladaptive: Interfering with an individual's activities of daily living or ability to adapt to and participate in particular circumstances. Repetitive maladaptive pattern: A recurrent trait–like repeat of earlier cycles and role-relationship models that, once clarified, can lead to reappraisals and growth, promoting learning in psychotherapy.
[6] Self-organization: A person's overall set of available schemas and supraordinate schemas.
[7] Schema: A usually unconscious meaning that can serve as an organizer in the formation of thought. Schemas influence how motives reach awareness and action. Schemas tend to endure, and they change slowly, as the integration of new understandings modifies earlier forms. Small-order schemas can be nested into hierarchies, together acting as larger-order or *supraordinate* schemas. Important types of schemas are *person* schemas (self, others, relationship), *event* schemas (marriage, etc.), and *procedural* schemas (how to do something).
[8] Therapeutic alliance: The relationship that forms between a patient and a therapist, allowing them to work together toward a mutual goal.

*Patient:* I find it embarrassing, but I could cry a river about my fractured marriage and divorce. But that is a "big over"; we ended 5 years ago.

*Therapist:* Sometimes it helps to follow the thread of your immediate feelings.

*Patient:* Ha, ha, doctor [in a sarcastic tone]. Got any CBT[9] techniques for quicker work on grief?

*Therapist:* I could agree to working as swiftly as possible when I know more about what's going on. You may want to avoid some painful feelings, and I wonder if a slowed-down conversation about them might make it tolerably safe—maybe not right now, but when you are in the sessions we have planned as a trial together.

*Patient:* Okay, starting over, I have been feeling heavy with a very vague sadness as if there is no future. [The conversation proceeds without sarcasm and with less avoidance.]

In this example, the therapist was observing the patient's verbal and nonverbal messages. They decided to ask the patient about a shift in their **state of mind**[10] by asking about emergent feelings signaled by the watery eyes. The patient had just brought up a heavy topic, the stress from the fractured marriage still present, but at the moment was in an avoidant state about their depth of grief, even though there was an intrusive breakthrough just before the avoidance. The aim of the therapist was to slow down the conversation, increase the patient's sense of safety, and so begin framing a sense of roles in a therapeutic alliance.

Initial individualized causal formulating is often focused on the possible interactions of psychological, social, and biological factors. In early sessions, the patient and clinician may select key problems and symptoms as targets for their work. They must consider what can change for this individual in view of personality features, social connections, finances, housing, and community structures. New events and changes in the patient lead to reassessments.

Usually, the clinician is personalizing language as they take a history. They observe how the patient spontaneously reports experiences, and they get detailed elaborations by asking questions. In addition to expert questions about history and symptoms, it helps to ask the patient about feeling in or out of control of the onset of a symptomatic state of mind.

---

[9] CBT: Cognitive-behavioral therapy.

[10] State of mind: A combination of conscious and unconscious experiences, with patterns of behavior that last for a period and can be observed by others as having emotional, regulatory, or motivational qualities.

Relationship patterns that may be maladaptive are especially important to observe and, when possible, clarify as possible topics for attention in therapy. This includes patterns of how a patient appraises themself and the therapist in different states of mind.

The patient's history includes past treatment. Additional information may be obtained through a mental status examination, record review, interview of collaterals, medical consultations as necessary, and the use of individually selected psychological scales. Patients seldom present without memories of prior professional opinions on their degree of mental health, possible psychiatric disorders, medications, spirituality, and psychotherapy.

Sharing realistic appraisals of circumstances is useful. These include aspects of the current setting, time limits, and the possible influence of third parties. For example, the patient may desire 1-hour sessions, but the therapist works in an organization that limits sessions to 45 minutes. Personalization has to take place in the present setting with its requirements and constraints, as therapist and patient try to reach initial agreements and discuss treatment goals and likely duration.

A clinician may use both structured and unstructured frames of discourse as seems optimum for the patient. A conversational style helps establish a therapeutic alliance. After each phrase is spoken or question asked, a clinician may listen attentively and calmly to how the patient reacts, elaborates, or avoids answering certain questions. Labeling a problematic topic in the patient's own words is a good way to focus.

Some patients will have doubts about (or unrealistic expectations of) what they can accomplish in therapy. A valuable technique for patients who overvalue or undervalue what they have been told by others or have read is to discuss frankly the therapist's skill set and knowledge base. In doing so, it is helpful to go beyond questioning to give feedback on what the therapist is thinking in response to what the patient has said.

Throughout the evaluation, the clinician seeks to clarify problematic themes. When a patient has had prior treatment, its effects and their relationship attitudes about prior clinicians may be discussed conversationally, as in the following example:

*Therapist:* How did your work with Dr. Smith end?
*Patient:* I just walked out on that doctor. He said I had been procrastinating at school.
*Therapist:* How did you react to him saying that?

*Patient:* So, I got your name.

*Therapist:* I get that sequence, but when you said you just walked out on Dr. Smith, it sounded maybe abrupt. I am guessing there were some feelings there.

*Patient:* You got wax in your ears? He criticized me! That's not helpful!

*Therapist:* I did hear you say that he said you were procrastinating. Perhaps that remark hurt your feelings? Perhaps you felt misunderstood? I don't know, but right now, do you mind my asking more about how you felt about yourself and about him?

*Patient:* I get it. You are not criticizing me. But I was irritated at him. Maybe for a moment at you.

*Therapist:* Yes, I can understand that. I wonder if there might have been some embarrassment at the idea of procrastinating?

The therapist thought that a useful pattern for future work may have been signaled by the patient's protest about the clinician's focus on procrastination. In focusing attention on the same topic, the therapist believes a tactful approach is indicated, using the words "maybe" and "I wonder" rather than saying, "I think you were embarrassed at the idea." This approach signals that the therapist is being empathetic and not at either extreme of accommodating too little to the patient's unease with the topic or accommodating too much to the patient's avoidance maneuvers.

Clinicians may work in an organization that requires a certain format for charting—sometimes the chart must be shared with the patient on a computer. Turning one's attention to a computer screen disrupts the conversational style. The therapist may also have to apply diagnostic coding according to the *Diagnostic and Statistical Manual of Mental Disorders* (DSM) or *International Statistical Classification of Diseases and Related Health Problems* (ICD) (American Psychiatric Association 2022; World Health Organization 2022). The patient may have had to fill out questionnaires such as the Patient Health Questionnaire-9 (PHQ-9) for depression. The conversational style provides an opportunity to find out about the patient's understanding of such frames. Any misunderstandings can be explicated and counteracted.

*Therapist:* You watched me when I paused and put some information about you into your electronic chart. What is your understanding of that?

*Patient:* What did you write?

*Therapist:* Some words you used for your main problems and some tentative impressions about what might be patterns or themes for us to focus on in the future of our work.

*Patient:* And some diagnoses so you can collect your fee by billing my insurance?

*Therapist:* That is part of how this department works. But this charting by typing onto a screen can feel distracting. It is required of me, but I also feel it as a distraction from beginning some useful work right now.

*Patient:* Yes, it is a bit annoying.

*Therapist:* I am glad you can say so. Yes, it can be distracting.

*Patient:* But I am not annoyed at you, just the machine.

*Therapist:* Me too, sometimes. But in the future you may feel annoyed with me, and I want to hear you say so whenever that is your experience.

The therapist's remarks are based on knowledge from psychotherapy research across modalities that a solid therapeutic alliance is an important promoter of progress in psychotherapy and correlates with good outcomes. Thus, they highlight difficult affects such as annoyance in advance of a patient's immediate intense experience. The phrase "in the future" is intended to create a safe alliance frame for what otherwise could lead to negative **transference**[11] and **countertransference**[12] reactions.

A therapeutic alliance is framed as different from and possibly containing transference and countertransference feelings. It has its own emotions, such as feeling pride or frustration in what is happening to promote the patient's long-range best interests.

Framing roles for each party in the therapeutic alliance, as modeled in the minds of each party (perhaps differently), begins during assessment. To bring such models into agreement, the therapist can request feedback and ask whether a sense of some accord is being reached as to the present process. An aspect of such a technique can be to ask frankly how a patient understands the clinician's role in the health system and the framework of interactions with the patient.

---

[11] Transference: Displacement of ideas, feelings, motives, and actions associated with a previous relationship to a current relationship, to a degree that the belief structure is, at least in part, inappropriate. In the context of a therapy session, when a patient unconsciously projects feelings from past relationships onto the therapist. Transference reaction: A state in which feelings are expressed that go beyond the frame of a therapeutic alliance.

[12] Countertransference: The opposite of *transference*; attitudes within a clinician that classically involve reactive feelings elicited by the patient's transference toward the therapist. Commonly, however, clinicians use the term *countertransference* to refer to feelings that the therapist has toward the patient, regardless of whether those feelings are brought on by the patient's transference.

Patients have their own expectations, and it is often useful to clarify them and describe how they may differ from how therapy proceeds. In most instances, therapy occurs in the context of some organization. Such organizations include practice teams, clinics, the enclosing health care system, and financial matters. In addition, patients have collaterals and current problems that affect their choices. This necessitates clarifying such issues as time constraints, session length and frequency, charting, online/telehealth options, and various insurance requirements such as prior authorization.

In these conversations, some emotions may be expressed, such as irritation at delays and limitations of the care system. The therapist's noncritical acceptance of such communications serves to establish a sense of mutual respect. Good listening, repeating what the patient says, and posing tactful questions gradually delineate the patient's needs, stressors, strengths, preferences, and social and cultural factors that limit their life.

This complex task need not be completed in the first session. It continues in later sessions and is revisited in stages of therapy after assessment. Therapy planning is also based on inferences about causal factors, not just diagnoses. This is an advanced goal that seldom can be achieved with completeness or certainty during first sessions. Most biological, social, and psychological factors interact, and the therapist may need to consider all these factors in the present transaction as well as how they occurred in the patient's development.

It is hard to get "enough" history in early sessions, and narratives about the past may not even be relevant in the evaluation stage. The technique is to start where you are and share that with the patient. It may be helpful to separate topics with fuzzy boundaries (fuzzy to allow consideration of interactions).

**Formulation**[13] is a continuing process, as will be discussed in Chapter 2 ("Formulating"), and goes beyond descriptive diagnoses as in DSM (Eells 2007; Cabaniss et al. 2011). Nonetheless, recordkeeping often involves recording diagnoses and may require a formulation. Formulation has the following components:

- A *case formulation* usually includes the biopsychosocial factors that have led to this particular syndrome in a person.

---

[13] Formulation: A summary of how a constellation of factors might be the cause of a syndrome that is also being defined by the interactions of these factors.

- A *personalized formulation* is one that pertains to this individual, with a focus on the current interactive factors.
- A *causal formulation* includes past as well as present factors.

The more complex formulations that occur later on will elaborate on factors that may include entrenched tendencies that lead to states of irrational shame and low self-esteem. Expectations of rejection or failure can lead to isolation, economic hardship, and career stagnation. Prior stress events such as loss, insecure **attachment,**[14] and adverse childhood experiences may be preconsciously expected to recur again and again. Being "stuck" in pathological patterns can also be caused in part by lack of neuroplasticity and thus limited connectivity between brain circuitries. This can be manifested clinically by a patient's poor reflective capacity.

In some settings, charts are open to patients. If the patient reads a case formulation, the clinician may offer elaboration, separating topics by focusing attention on "five Ps": presenting complaints, predisposing factors, precipitating situations and events, perpetuating conditions, and protective factors (Henderson and Martin 2014). Ambiguity must be tolerated in some of these topics, especially the issue of predisposing personality characteristics.

Personality traits stemming from a history of adverse childhood events may be of especially high importance in determining a patient's current capacities. Childhood traumas, losses, and exposure to structural prejudices can lead to excessive threat sensitivity and impaired control of emotional impulsivity patterns in relationships, dissociations of identity, and vulnerability to deflations in self-esteem. The therapist may discuss with the patient patterns that seem repetitive and maladaptive. Sharing hypotheses may help reduce the patient's pessimistic beliefs about the inevitability of a poor quality of life.

Conversations that occur during assessment may highlight topics, memories, and fantasies that are important to revisit in later stages of therapy. Agreements about where to start and what to postpone help establish a therapeutic alliance. In most psychotherapy, sessions include a therapist both asking, "what do you want to talk about today," and

---

[14] Attachment: A bond between self and other that is likely to endure. This term is used in formulation to refer to early bonds, perhaps established in the first 18 months of life, that may lead to a template for *secure, insecure/anxious, avoidant,* and *disorganized* schematizations of self with a potentially caring or abusive other.

suggesting, "maybe we can discuss more on [topic]." The aim is to share decisions of the therapy dyad's focus, now and in upcoming sessions.

The alliance characteristics of a typical assessment stage are summarized in Table 1.1. Reassessment will recur during support and all later stages of therapy.

## Support

Support begins during a skillful assessment. Listening closely and conveying understanding increases the patient's sense of safety during emotional experiences in sessions. The pattern of messages, verbal and nonverbal, going back and forth between therapist and patient builds a structure of roles and transactional patterns of a therapeutic alliance. Such alliances provide an expectation of safety, even when negative feelings are expressed. This growing, personalized relationship schema is the major factor in fostering positive change in psychotherapy (Stricker 2010).

The concept of personalized therapy means figuring out how quickly to promote expressions of the negative emotions that have motivated patients to begin treatment. A general technique is to stabilize rational states of mind in which the patient feels in some control, even of intense feelings such as grief. Some patients can go directly into intense communications of difficult feelings, but many need a period of extended support.

A supportive stage may include teaching techniques that stabilize states of mind and increase emotional self-control. For example, breathing techniques, body scanning, slowing down in a mindful way, and muscle relaxation promote calming and focusing on the present, factors that can reduce the frequency and intensity of anxious states of mind. CBT for insomnia may be indicated if the patient has complaints about their sleep patterns. Advice on finances, living arrangements, healthy nutrition, and exercise can improve general capacity.

The duration of the supportive stage may need to be increased for patients with personality disturbances. Regardless of the patient's level of functioning, however, the therapist can model realistic thinking while helping the patient understand how to communicate positively with others. Translating self-deflating attitudes into words and then offering alternatives is a valuable technique at this stage.

Problem-solving usually requires an understanding of the patient's family, workplace, culture, and racial, ethnic, gender, socioeconomic,

Table 1.1 Assessment stage of psychotherapy

| Patient activity | Therapist activity | Therapeutic relationship |
| --- | --- | --- |
| Report events, precipitating symptoms, problems, and preferences | Obtain history; make tentative formulations; provide information on treatment indications and options | Agree on initial frame of roles for a therapeutic alliance |

and educational characteristics. Impediments such as socioeconomic hardship, insecure housing, malnutrition, and lack of exercise can be addressed. Questions about specific self-deflating attitudes associated with any of these factors further inform what the therapist gleans from the psychological history obtained during assessment.

It is vital to establish and maintain clarity about the respective roles of the therapist and patient at this stage. Support provided in a therapeutic alliance is different from socializing or indulging in a positive transference enactment. Loneliness, isolation, and lack of constancy in social connections are common perpetuators of anxious and depressed states of mind. In need of some type of restorative relationship, patients may desire a *social relationship* rather than a *therapeutic alliance* with the clinician.

At times, patients may have feelings from activation of positive or negative relationship schemas. For example, a patient may idealize the clinical expertise of the provider. Then they become disappointed because the therapist does not provide "magical" support and remedies. A negative transference relationship model may take over for a moment, and the patient may be accusatory or angry. The technique that is generally useful in restoring a sense of therapeutic alliance is a calm response with tentative suppositions about why the patient has negative feelings. A calm demeanor shows that the therapist is not responding with fear, hostility, or guilt. Then the clinician suggests realistic possibilities for therapy to work.

Sometimes patients who fear abandonment by the therapist present a cold and aloof demeanor as self-protection. Sometimes patients worry obsessively that they will fall short in therapy and disappoint the therapist (Silberschatz 2017). The therapist may recognize these preconscious relationship expectations, and when they proceed professionally and do not respond with any negative messages to negative transference testing, the patient may feel safer, and the therapeutic alliance is enhanced.

For example, a patient complains that his depressed mood increased after members of his close-knit family ridiculed what he was wearing. He thought they shamed him because they didn't consider his clothing gender appropriate. The therapist said that reactions to this repeated humiliating situation might be usefully clarified by talking about it in therapy. Labeling the memory as a humiliating experience positioned the therapist as being noncritical and allied with the patient.

Clinicians can return to supportive techniques whenever needed. With support in place and some level of trust established, the therapy can proceed into a stage of deeper exploration of the meanings associated with key problems and symptoms. The characteristics of a typical supportive stage are summarized in Table 1.2.

## Exploration of Meanings

Assessment and supportive stages of therapy reveal emotional topics, maladaptive social patterns, and traumatic memories that may require deeper investigation. Enhanced expression and consolidation of fragmented memories can then occur in a stage of *exploration of meanings*. Associational connections between beliefs and feelings are clarified. Upsetting events, fearful expectations, blighted hopes, and **obstacles**[15] to goals are reviewed to promote realistic thinking and improve emotional regulation.

Counteracting defensive avoidances may be a useful technique in this stage. Sharing an observation—of a shift into avoiding emotional messages or troubling meanings of an event, for example—can improve an alliance if done tentatively and tactfully. A dose-by-dose conversation can be advised as a safe way to tolerate negative feelings. If the therapist shifts techniques from support stages to encouragement of more emotional expression and exploration of the motivations behind behaviors, this change in technique can also be explained.

For example, a 35-year-old man was in therapy for depressive and anxious states of mind triggered by current relationship conflicts. When he presented difficult choices about how to cope with a current plight, he frowned, knitted his eyebrows, and used vocal intonations

---

[15] Obstacle: An impediment to working through a difficult train of thought.

Table 1.2  Supportive stage of psychotherapy

| Patient activity | Therapist activity | Therapeutic relationship |
|---|---|---|
| Discuss current plights and problems; describe their ways of coping | Provide suggestions on how to improve coping and solve problems | Define each party's roles in promoting safety while discussing negative emotional states |

that indicated increasing tension. In earlier, supportive sessions, the therapist would summarize his recent set of remarks and suggest a possible, more-adaptive course of action. In the exploration-of-meanings stage, the therapist behaved a bit differently when observing the patient's state of mind shift to consternation and tension.

*Patient:* Now my dad insists I come to a dinner with his new girlfriend's family. Very bad timing for me but he's turning up the pressure. I hate him…no, I don't. Maybe I should just give in and sacrifice my other plans with Alice. [falls silent, stares at therapist, expecting a suggestion of what to do]

*Therapist:* [silently nodding in a way that signals acceptance]

*Patient:* Am I not talking about the right topic?

*Therapist:* I know I am being quiet. It is because I am waiting to see if you have any additional thoughts and feelings about what we are discussing. If so, we both might wait for those ideas and feelings to be spoken. What do you think?

*Patient:* I guess so. I am sorry I said I hate my father; actually, I… [continues on this theme]

With repetitions of this kind of remark, the therapist was able to promote a broadening of attention that helped to clarify underlying conflicted patterns. These had to do with behaving submissively to authority figures while feeling a confusing inner mix of anger, fear, and shame. The enriched alliance that was established during the supportive stage allowed the patient to feel safe exploring some ideas leading to maladaptive degrees of both resentment and self-criticism.

The frame of a typical exploration-of-meanings stage is summarized in Table 1.3.

**Table 1.3  Exploration-of-meanings stage**

| Patient activity | Therapist activity | Therapeutic relationship |
| --- | --- | --- |
| Expand on meaning to the self of stressful memories or threatening expectations about pending situations | Clarify how emotions and ideas are linked to symptomatic states of mind and maladaptive patterns | Discuss where to pay attention; deepen therapeutic alliance by maintaining a secure relationship during negative emotional expression |

# Re-narration

Assessment, support, and exploration of meanings may be sufficient to restore lapses in social functioning. For many patients, work in additional stages is indicated to modify entrenched maladaptive patterns. Therapy may progress to re-narration of personal stories from recent stressor events and from early life. Adverse childhood events may be reviewed and understood more realistically using adult thinking and reality-fantasy checks as shared with the therapist. Erroneous beliefs can be clarified and challenged by the therapist.

As memories are reviewed, the therapist can be alert to (and ask the patient to pay more attention to) the emotions of self and of other—in the memory, and in the present moment of review and reflection. Emergent anxiety or avoidance should be highlighted and the relevant passages of conversation reconsidered. This may lead to memory consolidation of a clearer story. It may also clarify insecure patterns of attachment, in which case the stages may advance to deeper work of re-schematization.

# Re-schematization

Re-schematization is the process of altering **belief structures**[16] by adding new elements, reorganizing prior elements, and altering linkage-strength patterns in the associational connection between elements.

---

[16] Belief structure: An associational pattern that connects elements of information into a meaningful complex.

The result can modify personality-based attitudes and assumptions. An important aspect of this stage is work to modify maladaptive self-other models, the basic scripts organizing relationships in various states of mind.

Schemas of self and other include **role-relationship models (RRMs)**[17] that function preconsciously as predictive codes of transactional sequences in repetitive maladaptive interpersonal patterns. These patterns are a recurrent trait–like repeat of earlier **cycles**.[18] The RRMs, if clarified, can lead to reappraisal and learning that promote growth. In most instances, they were developed in childhood and adolescence. When triggered, they can lead to social dysfunction.

Schemas may be unconsciously associated with a **psychodynamic configuration**[19] that can be gradually formulated. A configuration of conflict usually involves a wishfully impulsive aim, a threat that is viewed as a possible consequence of impulsive action toward a desired goal, and a defensive posture that, although it compromises the wish, avoids the feared consequences. A defensive maneuver may involve **reaction formation**.[20]

During re-schematization, techniques may include interpretation of some parts of a wish-fear-defense configuration. These may gradually be shared with the patient, and it may be helpful with some patients to start with **self-concepts**.[21] For example, self-images of being unattrac-

---

[17] Role-relationship model (RRM): An inner script or blueprint of interpersonal transactions, as well as attributes of self and others. Some RRMs are *desired*: they depict positive outcomes that a person seeks to achieve. Other RRMs are *dreaded*: they depict negative outcomes that a person seeks to avoid. In addition, some RRMs are *compromises*, used to avoid wish-fear dilemmas. Of these, there are *problematic* compromises, containing symptom-causing elements, and *protective* compromises, containing coping or defensive elements.

[18] Cycle: A repeated, sequential pattern.

[19] Psychodynamic configuration: A constellation of **motives** defined at the psychological level in terms of wishes, fears, and defensive strategies. A configuration of conflict usually involves a wishfully impulsive aim, a threat that is viewed as a possible consequence of impulsive action toward a desired goal, and a defensive posture that, although compromising the wish, avoids the feared consequences.

Motive: The reason for a decision. There may be motives to *enact* as well as to *restrain* action. There may be motives to think consciously or not to think consciously about a particular topic, memory, or unconscious fantasy. Motives usually refer to enduring themes in self-organization, whereas the word *intention* is used to refer to more transient aims.

[20] Reaction formation: The process of defending against one motive by augmenting some other motive or feeling.

[21] Self-concept: The recurrent belief of self-attribution that can be—and at least once, has been—consciously represented.

tive make it difficult to approach another person with a sense of worth and competence for interaction. Defensive withdrawal may be seen in terms of its maladaptive consequences: loneliness, depression, and certification of the deflated self-image.

It may help to call attention to progress, helping the patient feel more solid as a self and grateful for having their own source of inner self-esteem. Anxious and avoidant patterns of seeking closeness to others may be especially important to clarify and then interpret in a search for realistically thoughtful modification. Otherwise, the absence of mature models may limit capacities for social functioning.

Unconscious schemas that were formed during childhood may persist within disturbed attachment relationships and from experiences of trauma or neglect. Conscious **representations**[22] of schematic contents in conversations may be either inhibited or disturbing because of the activation of latent hatred, guilt, shame, or fear. Negative transference feelings may occur based on activation of some preconscious organizing schemas.

The feelings can be clarified in verbal conversations with the therapist. When the feelings are from transference, the therapist may interpret the difference between the activated transference model and the patient's new experience (in sessions, at times) of safe transactions of sharing and connecting in a therapeutic alliance.

Episodes of rupture of attunement and repair of a sense of therapeutic alliance can recur. The patient can learn better transactional scripts from **corrective relationship experiences**[23] within an enriched, resilient alliance. Technically, it may help to point out the repetition of a rupture, its triggers, and also moments of prior understanding of trust and containment of negative emotions in the safety of the best model of the patient-therapist relationship.

One aspect of such a technique is for the therapist to re-narrate prior moments in the therapy in which the patient felt deeply listened to, understood, and encouraged to express themself. Repetitions may improve self-attitudes, leading to a mature sense of identity featuring solidity and agency. Hope, purposeful goals for the self, and the ability to help others can increase joy in life.

---

[22] Representation: An iconic or symbolically encoded meaning that is capable of either conscious awareness or communicative expression. Representations occur in modes such as images, lexical (verbal) propositions, or enactive (somatic) propositions.

[23] Corrective relationship experience: A new transactional experience that builds trust and safety where distrust and danger have been entrenched as expectations.

**Table 1.4**  Attitudinal change through re-narration and re-schematization

| Patient activity | Therapist activity | Therapeutic relationship |
|---|---|---|
| Express ideas with emotions while talking about themes previously avoided | Help the patient modify dysfunctional beliefs and develop realistic memory sequences | Experience and remember new patterns of a secure therapeutic attachment |

Table 1.4 is a summary of the stages of re-narration and re-schematization.

Across stages, interpretive techniques can help a patient learn ways to increase executive functioning through more awareness of thoughts and feelings, better **insight**,[24] and more realistic choices on what to express to others. These processes lead to wiser relationship attitudes, as summarized in Table 1.5.

The following case example illustrates how stages of therapy can advance.

### Case Example: Teresa

In the assessment stage of therapy, Teresa said she was motivated to seek help because of a terrifying episode in which she felt a flood of uncontrolled rage toward her husband of 10 years. She and her husband had been arguing about household chores. She had become intensely angry and overreacted by screaming at him. He was shocked by this behavior, and so was she.

She was surprised by the feeling of hatred that she had toward him during the episode and feared that their marriage might end. Teresa had been having negative feelings toward her husband for months, but this episode was the first time that she had lashed out at him in an uncontrolled manner.

In the supportive stage of therapy, Teresa's anxiety about lack of self-control and a sudden marital termination was addressed as a prominent problematic state of mind. When she felt waves of rage toward her husband, or anxiety about a potential divorce, the therapist encouraged

---

[24] Insight: A realization about the cause or effect of a situation or a conscious connection between elements in a pattern.

Table 1.5   Awareness, insight, and new decisions

| Category | Awareness | Insight | Decision-making |
|---|---|---|---|
| Self-states | Knowing when a change in mood occurs | Understanding how and why a change in mood occurs | Planning how to handle triggers for entering problematic states |
| Altered unconscious controls | Recognizing inhibitors | Realizing why avoidance occurs | Choosing to focus attention on previously warded-off topics |
| Attitudes | Verbalizing views of self and other | Finding differences between old and new concepts based on new experiences | Choosing and rehearsing new schemas and scripts for social transactions |

her to use in-the-moment techniques to moderate her blame toward him. These included early-warning preparation by observing impending triggers. She could use momentary distractions for calming, breath control, and focus or walk away before she acted too aggressively with him.

She could also use pauses in therapy if feelings became too intense during discussions with the therapist and then go on after a respite. Teresa felt connected and normalized as the therapist reflected what she had said in a calm and clear way—for example, saying, "Many people get upset with people they love."

As the exploration-of-meanings stage expanded, Teresa was able to recall and recite memories of the marital relationship in a way that she could review with reality-testing types of thought. Teresa felt hopeful of increasing understanding as she talked. She and her husband had had a generally satisfying relationship for years. They had chosen to not have children and to each focus on their own career. Her husband had a successful professional career, and she owned a small business. Although they both produced incomes, her husband made much more money than she. Teresa felt less important than her husband and lucky that he had married her.

As the therapist and Teresa explored meanings together, Teresa put into words her patterns and beliefs, such as, "I must be with a successful husband to be a worthwhile person" or "I must never express my anger or I'll be rejected." When these beliefs emerged, the therapist helped her compare them with alternative concepts.

In the re-narration stage of therapy, Teresa was able to reappraise episodes with her husband realistically, rather than with thoughts of being undeserving and not entitled to self-respect. For example, the precipitating rage had occurred during an argument in which she interpreted her husband's comments to suggest that she should consider doing more of the chores because he brought in more money. She realized she did not agree with him and felt devalued.

As this theme of identity began revision in the re-schematization stage, she was able to see how she formed a model of herself that could be updated with her now more mature mind. As a child, her relationship with her father had been most important to her, but he always criticized her rather than celebrate her accomplishments. She was never good enough for him. She married a man whom she could boast about because he was so successful in his career. She was proud of being his partner, but she felt he did not feel the same about her. As a consequence of this model, she felt subordinate to his directions in their relationship, and that led to resentment—warded off, but eventually eruptive.

In therapy, Teresa re-schematized her self-organization, becoming more self-confident as she formed a competent adult image of herself. As she practiced balanced self-assertion, she improved patterns for intimate domestic partnership as well as tolerance for being alone, with growing esteem for her accomplishment. She told the therapist that they should plan to terminate after a few more sessions.

She had never felt safe discussing these attitudes with her husband. She felt ashamed that they were childish ideas. Feeling safer in exploring new attitudes with her therapist, Teresa came up with plans for herself, and she could speak of herself as worthwhile and independent. From this grounded stance, she could feel capable of being open with her feelings and needs and more assertive with her husband.

Later, Teresa reported that she was able to talk to her husband honestly for the first time in many years, and they were able to begin a process of renegotiating mutual goals and agreed-on responsibilities.

Inhibiting certain themes from clear representation had kept her from the lucid thinking that now led to more adaptive plans for various eventualities. With realistic possible paths and goals in the future, Teresa developed new self-schemas as a competent adult woman with a constant sense of self-agency.

**Table 1.6**  Drawing to a close

| Patient activity | Therapist activity | Therapeutic relationship |
| --- | --- | --- |
| Highlight gains and review future goals | Repeat the helpful new attitudes; clarify still-maladaptive patterns for possible future work | Emphasize agreement on when to stop, aiming toward a safe separation |

# Drawing to a Close

Eventually, the patient and therapist reach a point where they agree their work is finished. They have achieved the goals they jointly identified, and the patient feels equipped to carry on with the life they value. Drawing to a close rather than abruptly separating prepares the patient to leave the safe containment of the therapeutic alliance. This stage begins with reaching a tentative agreement some time before the last session is to occur. Setting this interval allows a review of the work that has made this choice possible. Options for future treatment, if indicated, are clarified. The termination stage is summarized in Table 1.6.

# Mechanisms of Change

Table 1.7 reviews the therapy stages.

# Summary

During the assessment stage, the patient increases knowledge of their condition and gains realistic hope as the frame for an alliance is clarified. During the support and exploration-of-meanings stages, the patient feels connected as the alliance increases safety. During stages of re-narration and re-schematization, the patient can think more realistically with the therapist and optimize models of self as transacting well in more satisfying relationships. In the end, the patient and therapist consider how adaptive changes may be maintained or advanced in the future.

**Table 1.7** Mechanisms of change

| Stage of psychotherapy | Mechanism of change |
| --- | --- |
| Assessment | Patient increases knowledge of their condition and gains realistic hope |
| Support | Patient feels connected and augments their sense of self-efficacy |
| Exploration of meanings | Patient connects chains of ideas realistically |
| Re-narration | Patient develops realistic appraisals of events |
| Re-schematization | Patient optimizes models of themselves in more satisfying relationships |
| Drawing to a close (termination) | Patient plans how to maintain adaptive changes |

## Key Points

- Every stage of therapy adds to the therapeutic alliance.
- A good alliance is a major promoter of morale, hope, and efforts to change maladaptive patterns.
- The therapist personalizes techniques by formulating causalities and sharing goals with the patient.

# 2

# Formulating

The goal of formulating is to explain why a patient has current dysfunctions and how they might be able to change. Early formulations are tentative and often lack understanding of deep motivational structure; the process deepens through stages of therapy. It helps to identify a patient's strengths, executive cognitive capacity, and sources of distress.

Previous formulations will have ambiguities and errors that can be modified as therapy progresses. That is why we talk about formulating, rather than formulation—an active rather than static process.

As we discussed in Chapter 1 ("Stages of Psychotherapy), in the early stages of therapy, the goal may have been to decrease symptoms. Subsequently, this goal may have been enlarged to modify entrenched maladaptive patterns. Formulation may have followed requirements for recording diagnoses and inferring biopsychosocial causes for the criteria symptoms. Entrenched maladaptive patterns may not have been identified in those assessment inferences. The therapy goes forward through stages, formulating these patterns as understanding proceeds from surface to depth, in a personalized way for each patient.

## Configurational Analysis

A states-of-mind approach is especially useful in such formulating and in personalizing treatment, because the patient's symptoms and patterns of interpersonal action may not exist in every state in an individual's repertoire. One method of formulating is called **configurational**

**analysis (CA).**[1] This approach to understanding a patient goes from describable moods to a depth of schematic structures and emotional potentials, including motivation. CA comprises four components specific to each patient: 1) **phenomena,**[2] 2) states of mind, 3) topics of concern, and 4) **self-other schemas.**[3]

These components of CA were developed empirically from research studies that reviewed video-recorded therapy sessions and assessed how to reach reliable agreements between clinicians (Horowitz et al. 1997; Horowitz 1987, 1991, 1997, 2005, 2011, 2019). The system is called *configurational* because it can clarify constellations of wishes, fears, and defensive avoidances as well as configurations of self-scenarios involving positive and negative social transactional scripts. That is, even regarding a given type of problem, the patient may have complex and not necessarily conscious associations between motives for happiness and safety, fears of becoming disconnected from belonging, and defenses such as social isolation and the illusion of self-sufficiency. CA helps the clinician observe and respond to changing phenomena while clarifying how to increase a sense of safety and reduce the imperatives of excessive **emotional control**[4] to avoid **undermodulated**[5] states of mind.

The surface component of CA is called *phenomena* because it describes the patient's complaints, symptoms, and signs in a personalized way, rather than as diagnostic criteria. *States of mind* are described as patterns of experience of emotions and expressions. The states-of-mind component helps therapists and patients share and clarify issues of variation in emotional valences and control. Observation of a shift into an undermodulated (or emotionally avoidant) state can include the *topic* (the set of ideas) that triggers the state change. Gradually, the *self and relationship schemas* that organize the experiences of different states of mind are inferred. Table 2.1 summarizes these components in relation to useful therapist actions.

---

[1] Configurational analysis (CA): A system of formulation that describes 1) phenomena to be explained, 2) states in which the phenomena do and do not occur, 3) themes that lead to state changes and defensive controls that are used to regulate the emotions of these themes, and 4) configurations of self-other attitudes.

[2] Phenomenon: An observable and reportable aspect of mental life, communication, and behavior.

[3] Self-other schema: Preconscious coding of the characteristics of each party and the expected transactions between them.

[4] Emotional control: Mental activity, often operating unconsciously, that wards off dreaded states such as anxiety, terror, rage, or depression. These regulatory processes use inhibitions and facilitations that can affect both form and content of thought, as well as schemas used to organize thinking, feeling, planning, and acting.

[5] Undermodulated: Observed to have lapsed in emotional control and contained regulation.

**Table 2.1** Configurational analysis

| Component | Purpose | Key aims for therapist |
|---|---|---|
| 1. Phenomena | Select symptoms and problems | Educate patient about symptom formation and techniques for mitigation |
| 2. States of mind | Describe states in which the symptoms do and do not occur; include states of avoidance and numbing of feelings | Help patient accept feelings instead of pushing away emotional experiences |
| 3. Topics of concern | Describe topics that evoke problematic states; describe excessive defenses | Clarify and challenge irrational beliefs and help patient plan effective action |
| 4. Self and relationship schemas | Infer roles and transactions of self and others for each recurrent state | Help patient learn adaptive attitudes for stable attachments and self-regard |

# Phenomena

Phenomena are reconsidered throughout the course of psychotherapy. Patient and therapist can discuss expectations and how to evaluate improvements. Techniques include educating the patient on knowledge in the field about the specific phenomena and how to decrease symptoms or increase tolerance for them if distress cannot be relieved quickly.

Part of this educational technique is normalization, in which the patient's particular complaints and symptoms are validated as known, not-uncommon experiences. For example, 68-year-old Phil became suicidal when he felt he was losing his mind. He was hallucinating that he heard and saw his dog who had died weeks earlier. He believed that the auditory and visual images indicated early psychosis. Phil's first response to his hallucinations was to feel pessimistic. He was reassured to learn that such quasi-perceptual experiences were a common part of a grief reaction. Education combined with the clinician's positive demeanor helped Phil regain optimism. He felt he could learn to tolerate his grief.

The therapist discusses with the patient symptoms and problems they want to change and what capacities they want to strengthen. The patient's answers indicate their degree of insight and motivation. These discussions can identify triggers for symptoms.

## States of Mind

The clinician discusses with the patient the states of mind in which symptoms and problems do and do not occur. A state description includes mood and degree of emotional control. Naming states helps the patient observe their own shifts in states; individually selecting labels helps focus attention; and having a shared label for a repetitive maladaptive state helps the patient anticipate triggers. Habitual defensive styles of avoiding explorations of meaning and emotion may be identified and given a label to help the patient in future self-observation. In this way, the clinician and patient can both comment on how qualities of affect regulation vary from state to state.

For example, Laura called her avoidant state her "tra-la-la" state and her mean-spirited, lashing-out state her "blue meanies." Laura and the therapist then found this shared understanding of labels useful to understand triggers for these two states and to identify alternative ways of expressing emotion.

A wish-fear-defense **configuration**[6] that is near the surface can describe the individual's repertoire of desired, dreaded, and avoidant states. After the murder of Laura's brother, Laura had attended the funeral along with her siblings and parents. Most were somber, but Laura expressed states of gaiety during the funeral. In her defensive state of gaiety, she seemed to exhibit denial of a dreaded, potentially intense grief over the loss of her much-loved sibling. Afterward, Laura suffered ongoing criticism during phone calls with relatives.

Laura described how she had expressed fake gaiety as being in her "tra-la-la" state. She was joking in a way others found inappropriate. During therapy sessions, she and the therapist came to understand the contrived humorous state as a defense against the undermodulated state of grieving—body-wrenching sobbing—that emerged in sessions.

Her grief felt out of control (hence embarrassing). In therapy, she gained **well-modulated**[7] states for owning and discussing her grief and the shame she felt when criticized by family members. On the way

---

[6] Configuration: A set of associatively related beliefs. Harmonious configurations have well-integrated elements, and conflictual configurations have poorly integrated elements, which can be associated with identity disturbances.

[7] Well-modulated: Emotion is appropriately expressive or contained.

to insight and understanding, she expressed the medley of unpleasant emotions she felt, such as sadness, guilt, shame, anger, and fear of future contact with the family.

Useful, general terms for clinician observation can include well-modulated, **overmodulated,**[8] or undermodulated. In addition, it is sometimes useful to note **shimmering states,**[9] in which the patient expresses an emotion and quickly acts defensively as if to cancel it. Evidence of the emotion is fleeting. For example, a patient who talks of the death of a loved one may start tearing up and then blink away tears, look away, stop, and then resume speaking tangentially.

Observing shifts from well-modulated states into under- or over-modulation helps a therapist (and then a patient) understand the effects of surges of feelings and reactive emotional controls. They can put into words both the emotional experiences of a state and the degree of self-regulation over the intensity of feelings and impulses to action. Verbalizing the type and intensity of the emotion may help both parties note and clarify what ideas and memories evoke intense feelings. This, in and of itself, increases a sense of self-control.

## Techniques When a Patient Enters an Undermodulated State

In a session, a patient's emotions can become undermodulated, leading to sobbing, rage, or panic. When that happens, the therapist models calm by speaking clearly and tentatively labeling emotions with common words. The therapist may repeat frequently, add words, and reorganize the sequence of ideas leading to feelings. Such techniques help the patient to slow down and reflect back. As the patient repeats a train of thought and has feelings in a titrated manner, the repetitions give them a chance to reappraise meanings.

## Techniques When the Patient Has Entered a Shimmering State

As the patient struggles between expressing and avoiding emotions, it may be useful to clarify what the patient has said and then stifled. For example, a patient might have said, "Then she criticized me, and I felt...well, never mind." The therapist can say, "I noticed that you

---

[8] Overmodulated: Emotion seems to be stifled.
[9] Shimmering state: A state that both expresses and stifles—or takes back—expression.

started to share your reaction to that criticism and then closed down. I thought you may have wanted, just then, to avoid going on with the memory. Did it seem that way to you?"

## Techniques When the Patient Has Entered an Overmodulated State

Sometimes patients interrupt their own emotional experience because it frightens or overwhelms them. By sharing what they have noticed at moments of emotional blunting, the therapist can help patients observe themselves. (A therapist need not intervene if the patient has shifted into an overmodulated state as respite from a state of high emotional intensity—once equilibrium is restored, the patient will change back to a working state.) Once again, the patient is willing and able to bring up and experience emotions. If the patient remains in an overmodulated state, the therapist may ask open-ended and clarifying questions to help the patient reduce avoidance.

# Topics of Concern

For Laura, the death of her brother and the family funeral were topics of importance—they were also triggers of her state shifts. Naming her "tra-la-la" state helped her observe her avoidance maneuvers. Naming these topics in relation to the avoided affects was a valuable technique, leading Laura to explore these difficult topics, including the shame she experienced from her family's criticisms of her behavior at the funeral. She and the therapist explored the topics of concern in relation to her current relationships with family members and her own critical self-judgment patterns.

The clinician's aim is to help a patient consider a realistic appraisal. To identify the obstacles to completing a train of thought, the therapist may share observations of defensive moments and hunches about what is being warded off. In doing so, it is helpful to use tentative language (e.g., "maybe," "I wonder"). Then the therapist can support and tactfully encourage the patient to think more about the previously unthinkable.

A patient's repeated approach to and avoidance of the emotional core of a particular topic can clarify for the therapist an unresolved conflict in the patient. The therapist may attempt a **clarification**[10] so that the patient is able to reflect on the issue. At the stage of exploration of

---

[10] Clarification: A clear verbal statement of a pattern and a chain of events.

meanings, it may help to normalize and externalize the inferred intra-psychic conflict of the patient. Making statements of common conflicts in others may increase the safety of this approach. For example, "Many people in circumstances similar to yours feel a struggle between love and duty. Some struggle with living by their personal ethics and living in ways that accord with what they have been taught as conventional standards within a family or community." If this leads to a conversation, the patient's conflict and values can be clarified, perhaps in terms of relationship patterns and future alternatives to maladaptive ones.

## Self and Relationship Schemas

Entrenched maladaptive patterns usually lead to states with poor regulation of self-esteem, depression, anger, and anxiety because of disturbances in relationships. They are *entrenched* in that the patterns may be based on enduring schemas from the past. This book uses the integrative language of *schemas*; the same underlying structures have been called transference templates, internal **working models**,[11] and attachment models.

Psychoeducation can help the patient view patterns as role-relationship models (RRMs). RRMs are inner schemas and scripts or blueprints of interpersonal transactions, as well as attributes of self and others. Some RRMs are desired: they depict positive outcomes that a person seeks to achieve. Other RRMs are dreaded: they depict negative outcomes that a person seeks to avoid. Still others are compromises: they are used to avoid wish-fear dilemmas. Of these, there are problematic compromises (containing symptom-causing elements) and protective compromises (containing coping or defensive elements).

RRMs can be raised into conscious reflection by verbal representation—talking about the role attributes of each party and how they have a pattern of acting and reacting to each other, as a kind of script of expected transactions (Horowitz and Möller 2009). The patient learns how they operate according to models that have unconscious coding for interpreting self and others. These models have attributes of self and other and include expected transactions, as a kind of script for sequences. There may be different RRMs and transactive scripts for expectations of negative responses from others, as well as positive responses.

---

[11] Working model: The currently active schematic organization of beliefs, usually combining perceived information and information from activated, enduring schemas.

It helps some patients to learn that these RRMs preconsciously organize how well they process information about possible attachments and decide what to express in a relationship or to feel as pride or shame in self-evaluations. The therapist can postulate configurations of wished-for, feared, and defensive models of relationships, relating them to desired, dreaded, and emotionally avoidant states of mind.

For example, Laura's state of false gaiety was a defensive model for how to relate to her family. To stay connected, she enacted an attractive clown role to bring them together in joy and affection. The behavioral pattern she enacted did not lead to positive attention, however, but to a relationship model she feared, in which she was seen as self-centered and seeking attention at a time when quiet communion was indicated. In therapy, a realistically more desirable aim was identified: she wanted to have a relationship with each family member and to share grief at the loss of her brother in an authentic and mutually empathetic manner.

Schemas are implicit rather than explicit. They are based on **procedural knowledge**[12] rather than **declarative knowledge**.[13] During the re-schematization stage of therapy, inferences are gradually developed until the clinician can discern the qualities that characterize the patient's views for organizing social transactions. Conflicts in motives for self-expression and attachments to others can lead to repetitive dysfunctional social transactions such as relationship ruptures. By focusing on future possible rage, panic, or bad-choice episodes, the patient can prevent some patterns from recurring.

For example, a patient had clarified a pattern of retaliatory rage when their domestic partner brought up something about them in an irritated tone of voice. Arguments followed. The therapist wanted the patient to learn alternatives to blaming each other for the argument.

*Therapist:* Now that we have clarified this retaliation that leads to a disruptive mood in both of you, let's image a less damaging scenario of a possible future repetition, when [partner] criticizes your behavior.

*Patient:* I guess I could try to say more calmly that that kind of comment hurts my feelings … but [partner] will just continue tearing into me.

---

[12] Procedural knowledge: Know-how that can lead to automatic action sequences without the concomitant declaration of such knowledge in reflective consciousness, operating either preconsciously or unconsciously.

[13] Declarative knowledge: Beliefs that are consciously represented and can be communicated.

*Therapist:* I also guess that could happen. Maybe, before continuing the discussion with [partner], you could take a short walk or do an activity that would calm you. Once calm, you could offer to discuss the difficult topic.

*Patient:* Worth a try. Can you review that for me again?

*Therapist:* Sure.

Hope for the success of such individualized techniques increases morale, and that amplifies a sense of self-efficacy.

In deeper stages of therapy, formulating can include explicating patterns of attitudes about the therapeutic relationship. Consider the personalized RRMs of the patient and therapist already generalized as 1) a *therapeutic alliance,* 2) a *social relationship,* and 3) a *transference.* Issues of power, closeness, constancy, and boundaries may differ among these RRMs. The therapist can put these various schemas into individualized verbal statements to help the patient differentiate reality from fantasy and learn what is really going on and what is possible.

Formulating may gradually expand to include developmental hypotheses about how, when, and why particular RRMs were formed. Attachment models, which are preconscious schemas of self as connected to significant others, may explain transference feelings such as separation anxiety based on core schemas developed from an insecure attachment in childhood. Identity may range from coherence to dissociative disturbance because of the presence or absence of damage from adverse childhood events, such as neglect, abuse, or parental loss.

Therapy often evolves toward the goals of increasing self-coherence and relationship constancy. It is hard for most patients to examine explicitly how a self-critic irrationally appraises self-worth and how this appraisal may shift from state to state. It helps to have a language about self-organization to discuss this (Horowitz 2014) and differentiate levels of awareness about identity structure, both conscious and unconscious. That is, with each patient, the therapist develops a shared language for talking about such things as threats to self-esteem, memories of disrespect, and a sense of vulnerability.

It helps to expand conversations so that a patient can talk about their sense of identity and how it may vary as organized in different **self-states**[14]

---

[14] Self-state: One of multiple ways in which an individual has learned to experience identity or to have an unreal depersonalization.

by activation of different nonconscious **self-schemas**.[15] A sense of identity includes a conscious belief that may be symbolized in words or images or communicated through bodily attitudes such as posture, gait, muscle tension, and gestures. A *self-schema* refers to a set of associative connections about self. Self-schemas are complex and include scripts, future intentions, hopes or ideals for self-realization, and cultural values. Alternative views—and in some patients, dissociated views—can be clarified with shared labels, such as "your strong self" and "your weak self."

A sense of identity may be different in different states of mind. The goal is to learn optimal functioning with a coherence in sense of identity across various states of mind. When there are conflicts between alternate self-attributions, descriptors, or dissociations, it may help to infer how the current sense of identity may be triggered by the activation of a particular self-schema.

For example, a patient who was a colonel in the army had a sense of identity as a heroic fighter. In some states of mind, he may have felt strong and purposeful. In other states of mind, he may have felt frail and incompetent. He had underlying self-schemas that included the roles and activities of a courageous man and others that included the roles of a sickly boy. It helped him as he learned to observe which state he was in: he became able to control his interpretations of himself so that he could feel stronger (but not omnipotent or invulnerable).

People vary in how well they integrate their repertoire of self-schemas and understand their own states of mind. Such integration or harmonization depends on how well they have learned realistic and conceptual self-reflective skills for dealing with contradictions between parts of self. (This will be discussed further in Chapter 5, "Paying Attention to the Patient's Current Level of Personality Functioning.")

In relationships, a sense of identity is influenced by the reflection of self by others. Being alone can be debilitating and lead to diffusions in a patient's sense of self, a kind of depersonalization. In supportive stages of psychotherapy, the emphasis should be on guidance and psychoeducation about how to improve connections with others. Then, in stages of exploring meanings, entrenched and maladaptive interpersonal patterns may be clarified.

The therapist can delineate and challenge dysfunctional beliefs. A calm, persuasive technique can be used, as in, "I wonder if you believe

---

[15] Self-schema: One of several potential configurations in cognitive maps that, when activated, can serve as unconscious organizers of many features of the individual into a holistic pattern of thought, mood, and behavior.

that you are not a potential person of interest to anyone in your building, so you just avoid conversational opportunities. That limits you in achieving a goal of providing yourself with more positive social interactions."

During re-schematization, the therapist can further clarify and challenge the patient's dysfunctional social cognitions about relationship dyads. These include maladaptive chronic outcomes in self-evaluating the experiencing-self dyad—such as a critic part and a judged part of self. This dyad is one part of the self praising or shaming what the other part of the self has done.

The origin of repeated self-critical voices can be explored in childhood memories of scolding and punishment. Interpreting these developmental experiences as related to self-criticisms can validate the patient's more rational and adult parts of self. Validating and repeating more rational self-conceptualizations are key techniques.

The therapist can help the patient review memories of conversations that disrupted a relationship and imagine a positive communication to counteract the negative model of transactions. The therapist, with the patient, can role-play a conversation; in the "two-chair" technique, the patient changes roles by changing chairs and addressing the other chair.

The goal of the improvisation is to calibrate the degree of negative emotion and the level of accusation at which useful understanding and negotiation of new rules can occur. This enhances the patient's skills for reflective practices and provides a more adaptive schematization for how to ameliorate patterns of mutual blaming.

Therapists can listen for and ask for the patient's identity concepts, especially adjectives such as *stupid, worthless, dirty, mean, unattractive, selfish, clumsy, incompetent,* and *fake.* By helping the patient represent core beliefs in lexical thinking, or graphic diagrams, the patient may develop better self-appraisal skills. Cognitive-behavioral therapy (CBT) techniques of sorting out the evidence for and against specific beliefs are useful in patients who are able and motivated to cooperate with the procedures.

The experience and un-worked-through memories and fantasies from childhood adverse events such as traumas, losses, and community displacements can be related to current dysfunctional beliefs about self. This may help the patient learn richer adult attachment models. The therapist can help the patient revise outmoded expectations and make new action **plans.**[16]

For example, a patient may exhibit a maladaptive pattern of being excessively sensitive to rejection. Adverse childhood events, such as a

---

[16] Plan: An anticipated way of coping with stress and realizing positive opportunities.

relationship with a needed other who was remote rather than caring and supportive, could have led to negative self-schemas. The patient becomes panic-stricken in a relationship where the other is preconsciously seen as a necessary but rejecting parental figure.

The script (when made explicit) is, "If I seek comfort by connecting amicably with so-and-so, they will just turn their back on me, or be scornful, so it's best to suffer loneliness without adding embarrassment and shame." This puts into words the therapist's tentative identification of an adverse predictive coding that has been embedded in the patient's unconscious schema by prior relationship experiences such as insecure developmental attachments.

The therapeutic alliance allows the patient to tolerate negative feelings as a part of accepting the therapist's technique of clarification and interpretation. In a kind of **parallel processing**,[17] transference feelings (and interpretations of them) may occur. For example, a patient takes a therapist's attempt at verbalizing a schema-based pattern as if it were a criticism. The therapist can reiterate their unconditional noncritical attitude in a way that challenges the patient's dysfunctional momentary belief—which, in turn, is based on a developmental schema.

Concrete concepts stick in memory better than abstract ones. When a patient depreciates themself ("I'm hopeless"), it is too abstract to reply "you have to increase your self-esteem." The concept is more likely to stick if stated in more deliberate terms (e.g., "Let's discuss how realistic that statement is"). Over time, the therapist parses an analysis and reinterpretation of a repeatable memory into short statements.

A long-winded remark can go unheeded because it is too complex. For example, John tells the therapist that he regretted an argument with his partner, Henry. He says, "I'm so stupid!" and falls silent. The therapist says, "I think it is better for me to argue a bit with you than to nod my head as if to agree that you are stupid. You remember saying 'I'm ending this!' to Henry. What do you regret about saying that? What are you sorry about? What else might you have said? Who in the past called you stupid?"

This otherwise good interpretation is too long and complex for John to process. Asking about the past, while sometimes useful, can also sidetrack goals of the present moment (how to have more positive social experiences). In this example, John did not repeat what the

---

[17] Parallel processing: The simultaneous processing of information in relatively separate channels; for instance, a person appraises a current situation through emotional cognitive processing that is organized by both a competent self-schema and an incompetent self-schema. Parallel processing can yield divergent conclusions.

therapist said and did not consider any of the elements that the thera-pist suggested. Instead, John said, "Why did I do that?" Both fell silent. Then John muttered, "I'm just so stupid." For a moment, the therapist felt stalemated. They said, more simply, "When a person says 'let's end this relationship,' there is seldom just one motive and one reaction."

Some patients may be in a state of mind that precludes complex cog-nitive processing. They require smaller steps, slowed-down reasoning, more time, and short parsing of statements by the therapist (Horowitz 2016a; Lindfors et al. 2014; Mullin and Hilsenroth 2014). Chapter 5 ("Paying Attention to the Patient's Current Level of Personality Functioning") discusses this concept further.

### Sam: Confronting Binaries in Dissociated Self-States

Sam, a 28-year-old man, developed PTSD symptoms after being attacked and robbed at knifepoint. Among his intrusive and avoid-ant symptoms were dissociative self-experiences. In some states, he experienced trains of thought in which he was a strong person who triumphed over an evil person. In other states, he was a weak person, threatened by possible confrontations with strong assailants.

He reported that he had been repeatedly victimized as a child by an abusive uncle. He recalled that, during the episodes of abuse, he had out-of-body experiences, seeing the assault happening as if he were on the ceiling looking down at himself on the bed. After the recent mugging, these memories became episodic intrusive images and dep-ersonalization experiences. Intrusive flashbacks of the mugging and fragmentary images of his childhood assaults continued for 6 months along with states of feeling himself to be unreal, "empty inside and not quite a person." He reported daydreaming of a future in which he was being killed or was killing an imagined attacker.

Formulating Sam's states of mind involved defensive **reversal of roles**[18] from weak (self as a victim) to strong (as in fantasies of kill-ing a perpetrator). There was no resting place. Strong concepts of self were too destructive and weak concepts of self were too fearful—hence the flip-flop back and forth. In therapy, this reversal was noted as a quick and confusing shift. The therapist repeatedly clarified what had been observed to happen in the sequence of discourse. The oscillations

---

[18] Role reversal: The process of shifting roles for self and other to defend against unwanted self-attributions.

between two extreme self-attributions could be expected to repeat. The therapist suggested that the two of them pay careful attention, striving to notice the moment of a shift.

With repeated clarification by the therapist, Sam learned how he shifted back and forth between different schemas. He could say how and when he shifted as he categorized himself as either too strong (critical, irritable, and punitive) or too weak (timid, withdrawn, submissive, and fearful). There was no room in between these two self-categories, which were segregated and implicit self-schemas with dissociated attributions. The goal was to make them explicit and harmonize them as parts of memory. The therapist described the goal as to find a unique, worthwhile self in the middle ground between extreme views.

The shifts from too-strong to too-weak self-concepts occurred with many topics involving both work and intimate relationships. As a particular memory was reviewed, the therapist and Sam learned to pay attention to shift points, moving from a self-appraisal as so strong as to harm the other person and potentially induce guilt to one as so weak as to be frighteningly vulnerable and ashamed of timidity. Then the therapist encouraged explicit, verbal reappraisals. In between the extremes, Sam might come to view himself as having new coping capacities. He could narrate about himself in the future as competent but neither super-strong nor super-weak in stressful potential situations.

To get to this middle ground, the therapist found it necessary to challenge Sam's present-moment dialogue. This sometimes meant saying that they were intervening to block the habitual switching. They might say, "Hey, hold on, listen to me, I think I hear you about to shift into telling me that you can be terrifyingly weak. I think you are giving up on what you were saying, which was how you are armed with strength, and this is that extreme kind of self-viewing we have noted. Anyway, that was the reaction in my mind just now. What do you think?"

At such moments, there were glimmers of transference feelings: Sam felt the therapist was attacking and criticizing him from a position of expert power. His tone and face were angry. At such moments, the therapist said calmly, "I am thinking that we have two things going on. One is you are attacking me for attacking you. The other is that I am not criticizing you and you know we stand together in trying to understand where you are. We are looking for new attitudes to change the switches between too strong and too weak. These are automatic thoughts, but we are working together to find new alternatives."

With lessened avoidance of emotional experiences, such as feeling frightened in public, Sam learned how to think consciously about his feelings and transactional expectations. He also learned how to think consciously about a middle ground between extremes. By thinking this way, he developed new scripts for relationship transactions.

In this long-term therapy, Sam became more able to converse reasonably. He would tolerate tension and fear without shifting back and forth between extremes of comporting himself as ragefully strong or shamefully weak. As he contemplated challenging topics and situations, he could remember that the therapist was tolerant of awkwardness. As Sam's capacity for **self-reflective awareness**[19] increased, his resulting insights helped him change.

When adverse childhood events have led to adult dysregulation of emotional expressions, sense of identity, and interpersonal behaviors, a systematic effort to augment tolerance of dysphoria and amplify emotional control is indicated. Through extended treatment, a continuous positive therapy relationship leads toward re-schematizing attachment models (Bowlby 1969), learning new social skills (Linehan 1993), and re-narrating memories of adverse events (Herman 1992). The therapist actively encourages the patient to see themself as an agent who can change their understanding of what happened and what may happen next (Greenberg 2011; Schauer et al. 2011).

# Relevant Theory of Mind-Brain for Positive and Negative Predictive Coding

Schema theory and its research basis are summarized in psychological terms in Horowitz's (1991) *Person Schemas and Maladaptive Interpersonal Patterns*. Neuroscience research has advanced theories of how the brain records and slowly modifies social schemas, as well as how brains may vary in capacity for understanding connections, attachments, and self-systems. Factors including genetics may affect a person's accurate or biased perceptions of self and others.

In terms of the kind of changes in self-other schemas that may occur during the psychotherapy stage of re-schematization, the patient's capacity for neural network plasticity is likely to be important. Complex networks of neurons are involved, with multidirectional

---

[19] Self-reflective awareness: A state in which self-observation is incorporated into awareness or sensory streams.

synaptic connections. Change requires complex alterations of both synaptic strength and connectivity. Of these complexities, the reward circuitry of the mesocorticolimbic areas of the brain is especially important, including prefrontal, nucleus accumbens, and ventral tegmental midbrain areas (Nicola and Malenka 1997). A change in circuitries could come from a traumatic abusive experience, leading to schemas that activate aversive predictive coding. New positive attachments, as in a therapeutic alliance, can counter with positive predictive coding.

Hypothetically, aversive predictive coding may be altered and reduced in circuitry functionality by establishing better schemas for expecting rewarding prosocial states of mind. Some experimental studies involve psychedelic-type drugs such as 3,4-methylenedioxymethamphetamine (MDMA, aka molly or ecstasy) and psilocybin, which may increase neuroplasticity, along with having powerful prosocial and empathogenic effects (Heifets and Malenka 2016).

# Frame of Attention in Therapy

For each component of CA, it is helpful to consider where the therapist should focus attention. Different frames may be segregated and compared, frames that vary regarding time and place. A pattern could be examined in terms of the present moment, in the therapy. If that pattern involves transference attitudes and feelings, then the frame may shift to the past, as in interpretations of developmental situations. Most conversations will deal with the patient's current memories of social situations. As already illustrated, conversations can usefully examine expectations and alternative predictions of the future in social situations. Table 2.2 summarizes this process.

# Process Notes

After a session, it helps to jot down process notes using CA. In notes on phenomena, a clinician can record changes; for example, "Insomnia improved from 3 to 6 hours of sleep on most days in the last week." In notes on states, the clinician can record observations of systematic patterns in qualities and apparent control of emotion; for example, "He was flat in emotional expression during the first half of the session, regulating feeling by intellectualizations and generalizations, but shifted into a working emotional state after I made supportive comments." In the session notes, under topics, can be recorded, "While he spoke

**Table 2.2** Components of configurational analysis and frame of attention

| Component | Frame | | | |
| --- | --- | --- | --- | --- |
| | Social situations | Therapy situations | Developmental situations | Future situations |
| States | Clarify triggers of problematic states | Teach how to share dialogue safely | Clarify emotional states during childhood | Plan how to prevent an out-of-control state |
| Topics | Counteract dysfunctional ideas and obstacles to emotional expression | Explore how and why emotional expression gets stifled | Re-narrate in adult terms the likely meanings of adverse childhood events | Plan how to negotiate with significant others |
| Self and relationships | Stabilize most competent self-images and enable restorative affiliations | Explore reasons for deflecting the therapeutic alliance | Explore evolution of self-judgmental values | Encourage enriched relationships and self-acceptance |

**Table 2.3**  Process notes

| CA component | Notes |
|---|---|
| 1. Phenomena: signs, symptoms, and problems | |
| 2. States: emotional qualities and control of emotional expression | |
| 3. Topics: themes and obstacles | |
| 4. Self and relationships: patterns and attributions of traits, roles, and intentions | |
| 5. Therapy technique: what I did and how the patient responded | |

of his indecision about whether to ask for a change of supervisors, he expressed his anger more clearly. That led to the state shift from flat to expressive." Under self and relationships can be recorded, "He called himself a stupid idiot who couldn't ever adjust." Under therapy technique, the clinician might write, for example, "I asked him who might have called him a stupid idiot as a child, and he recalled salient memories with both resentment and humiliation."

A block format for such notes is shown in Table 2.3. Readers of this book may copy or change it for personal use.

An overall configuration can clarify aims for technique and can be shared with a patient as understanding becomes more complex and feelings are verbalized in a safe manner, even when the experience is unpleasant. Common experiences of states and defenses can be stated in relation to goals for change. The perspective moves from past reappraisals to future aims.

Most people report periodic anxiety dreams (such as arriving in class unprepared or delivering a lecture in their underwear). The common fear is of shame emotions, and these may be reported in the pattern of actual maladaptive relationship transactions. As overmodulated, defensive states are reduced, these unpleasant feelings can be discussed in association with aims to develop well-modulated states, involving more pride in self and realistically assessing the self as a good-enough person and worthwhile to the community. These appraisals

Table 2.4 Awareness, insight, and new decisions

| Component | Awareness | Insight | Decision-making |
|---|---|---|---|
| Self-states | Knowing when a change in mood occurs | Understanding how and why a change in mood occurs | Planning how to avoid entering problematic states |
| Altered unconscious controls | Recognizing avoidance | Realizing how and why avoidance occurs | Choosing to focus on and rework previously warded-off topics |
| Attitudes | Verbalizing attributions of self and other | Finding differences between old and new concepts of self based on new experiences | Choosing and rehearsing new roles for the self |

are gradually established in conversations. Adaptive changes are highlighted by therapist repetitions in these conversations.

Psychoeducation can facilitate adult change away from repeating patterns derived from the past. This may or may not involve techniques for exploring childhood and adolescent memories of devaluation by similar-age peers or adults such as parents. The repeatedly clarified goal is to advance positive plans for productivity now that value to self and communities may be realistically appraised.

In psychotherapy, common mechanisms of change involve a combination of awareness, insight, and new decisions. State analysis with the patient gradually leads to a clarification of patterns in **identity and relationships**.[20] Insight involves self-reflection on key topics and feelings as well as defensive avoidances. New decisions can reduce defenses and other obstacles to therapeutic change. These aspects of working through patterns are summarized in Table 2.4.

---

[20] Identity and relationships: Schemas of self and others, including attachment models.

## Summary

An initial case formulation may include diagnostic issues and multiple causalities, such as biopsychosocial interactive factors. As therapy proceeds, so does the active process of formulating. Gaps are filled; ambiguities and errors are ameliorated. There is no conclusion, as the individual patient remains a person in motion in the midst of life and its vicissitudes.

## Key Points

- Formulating is an ongoing process of personalized understanding of the complex and often ambiguous biopsychosocial factors that have shaped the present situations and patterns.
- Sharing tentative observations with the patient can be a path of clarifying and considering what can change.
- A states-of-mind approach can help both patient and therapist focus attention on shifts, as in increasing or decreasing defensiveness.
- The therapeutic alliance allows the patient to tolerate negative feelings as a part of accepting the therapist's technique of clarification and interpretation.

# 3

# Choosing What to Say in the Present Moment

Listening deeply is a vital aspect of therapy. Done well, it includes attention to the verbal and nonverbal signals of the patient and the therapist's own internal mental experiences while listening. These observations include detecting the therapist's own small startle reactions (something different here, why did the patient just say or move that way?). Internal observations include incipient, possibly useful actions (is now the time for me to share what I think just happened in the conversation?).

It helps to learn ways to 1) remember the alerting observation, 2) formulate why the observation is noteworthy, and 3) anticipate what consequences of the therapist acting now might be. If an action is taken, then the clinician observes the effects, and the cycle repeats. This can lead to reformulating and revision of technique. Such a cycle in the therapist's mind is mostly intuitive, but a possible model is shown in Figure 3.1.

A common technique in therapy is to help the patient focus attention on a difficult topic. Clarification occurs in a back-and-forth dialogue, one that elaborates and connects meanings while regulating emotional intensity within safe limits. The therapist can appraise the process, calibrating whether a sense of cooperation is increasing or decreasing (because of increased defensiveness, for example). Usually, the most important alerting observation is that a patient shifts into an avoidant state of mind as a reaction to a therapist's action.

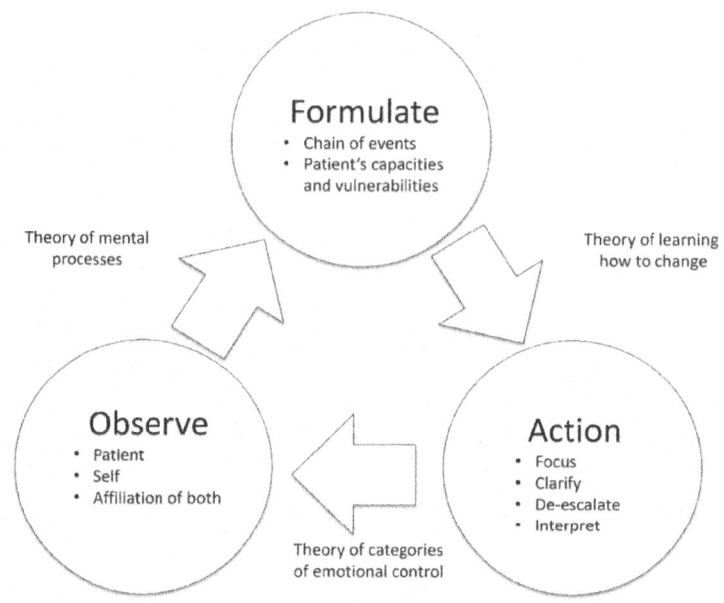

**Figure 3.1** The therapist's cycle of observing, formulating, and acting.

If that happens, the therapist might respond by saying, "I think you moved off that topic I just talked about as a useful way of self-calming." (Note the positive word, *useful,* is probably better than a negative word or phrase, such as *running away from.*) The support of being accepted, rather than criticized, reassures the patient that avoidances are normal.

Such conversational transactions encourage the patient to express what they were warding off. The therapist then observes to see if the patient enters a more connected transactional state. On the other hand, even tactful challenges to the defensiveness of a patient can lead to reactive anger expressed toward the therapist. Sometimes, the target of the potential feelings may be shifted from some other person to the therapist. That is, the target of feelings toward an unhelpful other may be **projected**[1] onto the therapist in a transference type of role-relationship model (RRM). If the transference feelings can be contrasted with

[1] Projection: A defensive operation in which an attribute of the self is externalized and regarded as coming from or motivating another person's perceived emotions, words, and actions.

the qualities that both parties can now observe in the actual therapeutic alliance framework, then a change in attitudes may be possible.

Such a present attitudinal change moment has several components. One component is the emotional activation of an old model for self-other that acts as a preconscious predictive coding and leads to transference expectations. This activation of an entrenched pattern leads to feelings such as anger because the patient preconsciously anticipates that the therapist intends to shame the patient. The patient reacts because of an expectation of criticism. The therapist's communications of empathy, compassion, and support counteract the patient's expectation of being embarrassed.

A useful technique is to clarify the old schemas and challenge them by explicit statements of the therapist's intent to be accepting, caring, and noncritical. This declares the experiential authenticity of a therapeutic alliance. The pattern noted in the emotional passages of a transference enactment may indicate anger at feeling belittled. The new information—how to carry forward a calm dialogue without mutual blaming—can be learned as a new pattern for future interactions.

If the archaic RRM activated in transference was derived from adverse childhood experiences, the new relationship experience is a corrective relationship experience because it is a second chance to learn how to form and sustain a secure attachment (Bowlby 1969). The secure base of the therapeutic alliance can provide the patient with courage and stamina for exploring various painful relationships. New guidance from the therapist can help promote the acquisition of new schemas (Brown and Elliott 2016; Horowitz 2016a; Young 1990). Later chapters in this book deal with these techniques in more detail.

How rapidly such learning may occur depends on a patient's current capacity to think logically. In a therapy that uses clarifications and interpretations as prominent therapist actions, the questions arise: Does the patient understand the therapist's meaning and gain insight? Does the patient have sufficient capacity for mentalizing both self and the therapist's intentions, which are in the best interests of self in the long run?

Techniques used in the hope of advancing identity concepts and relationship models often involve stating in words possible linkages between developmental relationship experiences and current maladaptive patterns. Some patients may not have the capacity to understand what the therapist means by these interpretive connections. When patients do not understand the therapist's intentions, they may feel invalidated or even assaulted, rather than safely accepted. Patients who function at a lower level of development require more time, tact, and parsing of statements by the therapist (Horowitz 2016b; Lindfors et al. 2014; Mullin and Hilsenroth 2014).

# Social, Therapeutic, and Transference Attitudes of Patients

The relationship frame, as offered by the patient, may shift during the session as well as between sessions. It is not uncommon for the patient to assume a kind of **social alliance**[2] in the opening moments, walking with the therapist from a waiting room or starting a remote telehealth session. Comments on the weather, politics, or sports may be amiable and jointly "human." The state of how the patient and therapist relate may shift in ways organized by the roles of a therapeutic alliance. Toward the end of the session, a social alliance frame may be restored, as the patient resumes "a social face" for self-presentation to the world outside the session.

For example, a patient may begin with comments on the weather, which are received amicably by the therapist. Then the patient may tell of a relationship dispute they are "stressing over." This represents a shift from social to therapeutic alliance qualities. Later, the patient gets angry at a message from the therapist. This may be a reaction to a transference feeling of being unfairly criticized. The irritable state from a transference framing of roles dissipates as the therapist's calm responsiveness helps the patient reinstitute the organizing RRM of their schemas for the therapeutic alliance.

A therapeutic alliance can accommodate many techniques, including playful ones, as in this example:

*Patient:* My heart is so broken!
*Therapist:* Your face does look very sad right now. That is a real feeling, and you are really expressing it, so I think that I do get an understanding; it is like I am sharing your grief right here and now.
*Patient:* Why did you say that?
*Therapist:* I said I thought you looked sad, and that your feeling message felt real to me, and my empathy said it might be grief. Anyway, your state of mind seemed unlike that "I don't feel real" state you spoke about earlier.

---

[2] Social alliance: A framework for roles in a dyad that is reciprocal and learned as a context for the degree of sharing of feelings and problems.

*Patient:* [smiling] So if I say I am worthless, a nothing, that is real?

*Therapist:* I think right now you're teasing me, and that's okay with me because it is playful. I think you know I was saying your feelings felt real to both you and me. I certainly was not saying you either feel unreal or you feel like a nothing, as if those two states were the only choices ahead.

*Patient:* [silently listening and looking at the therapist]

*Therapist:* You know, I think that the playfulness is part of learning how to get out of that state of fragile heartbrokenness.

*Patient:* Okay…I get it. I was kind of poking at you. But let me tell you why I got down in that blue mood of feeling worthless. [expands on a recent memory of feeling rejected by another person; describes how the other might have thought them unworthy of affection]

These three categories (social, therapeutic, and transference relationship models) are useful to keep in mind for observing the present moment. Social alliance is a concept that may help in understanding those moments at the start and end of sessions, when therapist and patient acknowledge the humanity of the encounter and fare-thee-well of separation. Sometimes observations may include awkwardness. When the time is right, this awkwardness can be addressed by the therapist in a personalized way, as in the following example:

*Therapist:* As we ended our last session, I noticed that you said goodbye to me in a way that struck me as very gracious. Afterward, I thought I perhaps seemed terse or short with you. That made me think that we may have a different community or cultural background on how to say goodbye for the time being.

*Patient:* Yes, we do. I know a little about you, and we look and dress in different ways. But you and I usually understand each other really well. A new thing for me. That reminds me that I was surprised when you did not agree with me that my brother should be told to criticize his wife for dressing immodestly at my birthday party. Didn't you agree with me?

*Therapist:* I remember. I was silent but not disagreeing. I did not mean my silence to signal disagreement with your values. I am glad we can discuss this now.

*Patient:* [somewhat irritated tone] Then what?

*Therapist:* Then, in that session, and right now, I want and intend to hear about your experiences, including feelings toward your brother, toward me, and toward yourself as a person with varied attitudes.

*Patient:* What is your attitude about modesty of dress?

*Therapist:* I want to expand my understanding of you in your various circumstances. I have much to learn, but I do feel it is important for me as a psychotherapist to have a multicultural orientation and cooperate with accepting differences in opinion and values.

*Patient:* Oh. I like that. [continues to discuss brother]

The point of this example is that the therapist is not afraid to hear that the patient knows the therapist may have a different background, alternate values, and some customs of engagement that are not symmetrical. Putting the specifics into words—agreeing on meanings and basic frames—leads to learning.

# Trauma

Trauma is rife in the public awareness. Processing of an adverse event such as rape is discussed in social media, movies, podcasts, and telehealth sites. Patients may want what they have seen in such settings—that is, they may want therapy sessions to focus attention on processing of childhood traumas that, in their opinion, have never been processed.

This public attention to trauma makes for special problems in personalized technique because review of childhood memories of abuse and neglect may not be the priority in the present moment, which perhaps should focus on current problems and choices for how to adapt. As I discussed in Chapter 1 ("Stages of Psychotherapy"), when the patient has experienced multiple adverse events, it may be beneficial to deal with present and future issues before going into deep formulations and memories of childhood adversity.

The choices of present-stage techniques do involve history and schemas of the present. Re-narration and re-schematization of trauma memory/fantasy scenarios can be helpful, or it can be re-traumatizing, leading to negative feelings and flash intrusions rather than improved well-being. It helps to experiment with time frames: the present, future expectations including plans and goals, and past experiences.

Because trauma is so prevalent in the news and social media, patients may benefit from psychoeducation about how the mind works for most people. One approach is to explain how trauma and loss events leave complex memories that may require processing involving multiple (and not necessarily well-connected) associations in different brain registries. Realistic appraisals and coping strategies may be impaired by automatic activations of irrational beliefs or immature understanding.

If that happens in therapy sessions, negative emotions of fear, rage, sadness, and guilt may threaten to flood and disorganize the patient's thoughts. Processing may be inhibited because of intolerance of the feelings evoked by recalling memories and fantasies or reviewing flashbacks. Unconscious avoidance intentions may prevent adaptive memory reconsolidation and adaptive coping.

Psychoeducational techniques may help a patient understand how their own mind has associations of meaning that are both compartmentalized and connected. The mind tends to repeat fragments of traumatic memory and fantasy until it achieves integration across circuitries and its predictive coding accords with the real world in the present. Personality traits and capacity for neuroplasticity affect repetitions and reappraisals, desensitizing intense automatic fear arousals. Therapy is slow (in spite of reports of sudden change) because the process of change is complex for everyone. In addition, people are different in how fast they can go through a slow process.

Disturbances or damage to executive capacity for thinking and regulating emotional intensities may affect symptom formation. Conversations in therapy can facilitate cognitive processing. A patient's enhanced control of emotion in the safety of a therapeutic alliance can reduce the extremes of intrusions and avoidances.

Every patient is affected by history. Cultural and economic changes impact all our lives. Childhood internalized values and beliefs from culture, community, and family tend to change from epoch to epoch. Even with some constancy of a patient's loved ones and spiritual teachings, there may be present-moment conflicts—for example, in the right and wrong ways to mourn and express grief.

To help tailor the treatment stage of working through trauma and losses, whether recent or from memories, phase-oriented techniques may be used, as well as psychoeducation on why the therapist is suggesting certain techniques. Phases in PTSD and prolonged grief disorder share variations from symptomatic extremes, from flooding with intrusive memories and emotions to avoidant states of mind (Cloitre et al. 2009; Horowitz and Möller 2009; Horowitz et al. 1997).

In earlier *denial* phases, inhibition of emotion leads to numbness, avoidance of reminders, social withdrawal, and distraction. Self-damaging avoidance may include disavowal of the implications of the event. Self-medication may lead to symptoms of substance abuse.

Underregulation of preconscious memories pressing toward repeated conscious representation shifts the state of mind into an *intrusive* phase. The individual may report unbidden flashbacks, nightmares, compulsive enactments, and flooding of negative emotions such as anger, fear, despair, shame, and guilt. Compulsive behavioral reenactments can occur, as can physiological exhaustion from chronic hyperarousal, with various somatic consequences (Horowitz 2011).

Immediate symptomatic responses include intrusive phenomena; likely to be addressed first are these symptoms based on fear conditioning: pangs of emotional distress with reminders (startle reactions, panic, sudden aggressions); physiological reactivity to reminders (tachycardia, startle responses); difficulty falling or staying asleep; and difficulty concentrating. Gradually, the patient clarifies and addresses these experiences to increase emotional control and reduce secondary fears such as "going crazy."

A patient's intrusive recollections may lead them to avoid conversations about traumas and activities, places, or people that provoke recollections of the event (phobias). During an intrusive phase, the patient may paradoxically be unable (through conscious intention) to recall an important aspect of the event. Oscillations into denial and numbing may occur. Apathy can lead to markedly diminished interest and participation in significant activities (social withdrawal and anhedonia). The resulting loneliness exacerbates the depressive state of mind.

It is important to address these intrusive states using whatever techniques help this particular individual. The patient's experiences of specific intrusive memories may be lessened through gradual desensitization and extinction, as in trauma-focused cognitive-behavioral therapy (CBT). Techniques for enhancing mindfulness (body-scanning, breath control, and meditation) may increase tolerance of unpleasant moods and experiences. Patients can supplement therapy sessions with online resources such as CBT for insomnia.

Maria, a 40-year-old widow, sought help after the death of her husband of 20 years. They had fought his cancer together for 3 years before he succumbed. She had anticipated his death for some months and thought she was ready because they had gone through a great deal of anticipatory grief. But Maria was surprised by the intensity of her symptoms. For weeks after his funeral, she experienced disrupted sleep, fatigue, frequent states of fearful agitation, and a sense of depersonalization.

She expected to tolerate loneliness and sadness, but intrusive images of his vacant eyes and an urge to "just do something to save him" occurred in her undermodulated state of mind. She was even more startled to feel empty, as if she were not a person. She described how she shifted from undermodulated agitation into a more avoidant, numb state of mind. This overmodulated state of mind caused her to conduct her life in a ritualized and anhedonic manner, as if not herself alive. She could not think of memories of being with her husband in that state. She was able to carry out domestic tasks, but she experienced no satisfaction and sought no conversations with other people.

The therapist took a psychoeducational stance and told her that this numb state was a way to avoid feelings that they might gradually discuss together in a safe way. People who have lost a loved one frequently experience painful states of feeling empty and numb, but also develop tolerance for loneliness and longing. The therapist said that Maria loved her husband deeply and missed him greatly. Right now, in some states of mind, she was not loving herself and was missing herself in a positive self-state, as reflected in the domestic interactions of that marriage. By setting therapy goals that worked toward changing her situation, she could eventually feel safe in trying for new and positive social connections with others.

Accepting expressions of negative emotions in the safety of a therapeutic alliance is a core process in therapy. The optimum communication between patients and therapists occurs in states without too much flooding or too much inhibition. The state-oriented technique aims first to stabilize rational, working states in which the patient is neither overmodulated nor undermodulated. The goal is to deal with emotions, motives, memories, and fantasies in conversations that feature rational reflection.

When the patient expresses intense affect and signals that they feel out of control, they are experiencing a repetition of intrusive phases. In such instances, as I discussed in Chapter 2 ("Formulating"), techniques that help are slow repetitions with explicit statement of intentions. That is, the therapist helps them slow down the rapid fire of thoughts and memory fragments, with an aim to de-escalate and tolerate emergent negative emotions. The therapist models calm by speaking clearly while naming the ideas and emotions that threaten to flood the patient's mind. The therapist shares what they have just observed, promoting reflection and understanding. Such clarification is not easy, and the therapist may ask the patient to correct the therapist's tentative appraisals.

Alternatively, it may help to repeatedly explain the value of frank, nonjudgmental communication of emotional ideas, call attention to specific moments of avoidance, and show how safety within the containing context of therapy makes it unnecessary to inhibit expression.

The therapist can continue to show how to explicitly label the avoided ideas and feelings.

Topics considered especially in re-narration stages of therapy are usually about memories and fantasies that have not fully consolidated the meanings of stressor events with other life stories. Often, a goal is to piece together memory fragments and connect otherwise dissociative elements. Many narratives of adverse events incorporate fantasy elements or vivid perceptual "snapshot" images. Most patients feel to some extent that their memories are incomplete.

Some techniques include memory fragment connection, while moderating anguish and impulsivity by verbally naming emotions and impulses, normalizing self-image with psychoeducation, and addressing comorbidity and social circumstances. The therapist may float a short story describing how events may have occurred. The patient responds with suggested revisions, and the back-and-forth conversation can be both a reappraisal and a desensitization experience.

As therapy progresses, more complex patterns can be explored, such as excessive self-blame leading to excessive shame, guilt, or self-disgust; excessive blame of others leading to easily activated rage; despair or suicidality from a sense of inevitable doom; self-disgust from a shift from competent to incompetent images of self or from attractive to unattractive; enfeebled images of self; and vulnerability to an annihilation panic state from a shift from coherent self to derealization and dissociation (Herman 1992).

One common topic is who or what is to blame for a stressor event. Blame that is directed outward tends to activate outrage and revenge fantasies (Horowitz 2021). Blame that is directed inward tends to activate guilt and shame. Defenses against self-disgust may include excessive projection of blame away from the self. Projection is a defensive operation in which an attribute of the self is externalized and regarded as coming from or motivating another person's perceived emotions, words, and actions.

Cultural sensitivity on the part of the therapist will help clarify the patient's theories of why stressor events occurred and who or what is to blame for harm or inadequate protection. Topics of religion and spiritual practices may be explored to clarify the patient's conflicting values. Techniques that reduce inhibitions and increase insight and self-reflective awareness include promoting lexical representations with an expression of feelings.

## Summary

Personalized and integrated psychotherapy is promoted by the therapist's actions. Choices of what to say and what not to say are optimized by understanding the complexity of the patient in the present moment. The therapist's technical abilities increase as they learn more and more.

## Key Points

- The present moment is about the relationship between patient and therapist; pay attention to connectivity (whether it is improving and empathetic).
- A useful alerting observation is that of a patient shifting into an avoidant reaction to a therapist's action.
- Strive to work on difficult topics during productive states of mind, using reality testing of attitudes that may have become ingrained maladaptive patterns of thinking.
- In the psychotherapy of trauma, it may be more important to focus attention on the present and near future rather than relive childhood adverse events.
- Once undermodulated states have been ameliorated by learning to tolerate negative emotions, the past can be re-narrated with an adult mind rather than a child mind.

# 4

# Techniques When Obstacles Stall Progress

As therapy progresses, a patient may observe that they have reduced intensity and frequency of undermodulated states of mind. That makes it possible to promote adaptational learning by discussing, in relatively well-modulated states, topics that are conflicted (Sloan et al. 2017). At times, during these deeper explorations, defensive obstacles may still episodically stall progress. If so, there are ways to counteract these defensive maneuvers so that a therapist may help a patient further modify their maladaptive ways of regulating emotion.

Habitual defensive maneuvers may have evolved from avoidance maneuvers that helped the patient during development (moving away from fears and reexperiencing memories of adverse experiences). The defenses that have become habitual can be replaced by learning new, more adaptive emotional regulation capacities (Aldao and Nolen-Hoeksema 2012; Aldao et al. 2010).

A generally useful technique is to take on only parts of hard topics. When the difficult ideas and feelings within a hard topic get represented, a patient may wish to "get it over with" rapidly. They recognize the theme, saying that now that insight has occurred, the topic is over with. Going back over one subtopic can help the patient continue with new insights on the habitually warded-off ideas and feelings. A therapist teaches how to slow down the patient's train of thought and allow smaller pieces of conversation to provoke shared reflection on meanings.

The technique of making open-ended remarks may enable the patient to engage in fuller emotional expression without an avalanche of too-intense feelings. For example, a 40-year-old patient and therapist were focusing attention on the patient's memory of a recent upsetting argument with his adolescent son. The patient, at this moment in therapy, was in an overmodulated state.

The therapist observed the patient avoid emotional expression by the (probably habitual) defenses of intellectualization, generalization, and quick closure of thinking or conversing on a topic. These defensive maneuvers seemed to the therapist to have a possible purpose of avoiding the emergence of a self-image as a bad father. The therapist decided to help the patient experience emotions bodily and label them in words while reviewing a segment of a specific recent memory.

The tentative formulation in the therapist's mind was that the patient might feel he had been too critical and wanted in the moment to avoid shame as a felt emotion. The therapist thought it premature to make any such interpretation. Instead, avoidance of anger in the story of an episode seemed a gradual approach.

From the context of what the patient had been saying, the therapist inferred that probably both father and son were angry during the argument. Instead of labeling that emotion as anger in direct words, the therapist decided to interpret what might be going on defensively.

*Patient:* I got upset when he argued with me about those things. So, then I went to the pantry for a snack. That's that, I guess. [silent]

*Therapist:* I notice that you started out by saying you were upset when he argued with you, but next you seemed to avoid saying any specifics about how that felt.

*Patient:* [stays silent]

*Therapist:* [also remains silent, looking at the patient with an expectant, calm facial expression] I guess I was thinking "upset" is a very general word.

*Patient:* Well, we were in the kitchen, and I was only a little bit irritated. Anyway, I am sorry about it all. Let's leave it at that. [silence again, looking away from the therapist]

*Therapist:* I am not sure, but am I correct in thinking your son had done something wrong? You were admonishing him, and then he disagreed with you, upon which you felt angry at him?

*Patient:* [angrily] No, of course, I was not too irritated with him!

This was not what the therapist was hoping for as a response. Instead, listening to the patient, the therapist believed the patient became angry at the therapist. The therapist inferred that the patient's moment of irritation was an avoidance of shame regarding the argument with his son. In other words, what the therapist formulated privately was that the patient, in the present moment of the therapy session, was preconsciously anticipating being shamed by the therapist for expressing too much anger at his son.

With this tentative understanding, the therapist thought that the patient was incipiently angry with the therapist for exposing him to potential embarrassment if he told the story in a way that expressed his degree of anger. The therapist chose to challenge the patient with a somewhat paradoxical reflection of what the patient had last said— paradoxical in that the therapist joined the defensive position rather than interpreting the angry feelings or the potential feelings of shame.

*Therapist:* Oh, so of course, you were not very irritated with him. I guess, maybe, he was the one who was angrier at you? [said in a matter-of-fact tone, not sarcastically]
*Patient:* I don't know.
*Therapist:* Maybe tell me more about your memory of who said what in the kitchen.
*Patient:* My son said I was wrong to ground him for coming home too late last Friday. I said he knew our house rules. He glared at me. I wanted to leave the room or yell. Yelling is bad; it is what my own father did too much. So, I wimped out and let him get away with it. I don't like that in myself.
*Therapist:* You don't respect yourself for either extreme, "wimping out" of fatherly duties or harming the relationship with too much forcefulness.
*Patient:* I would like to learn how to handle my surge of anger when that kind of thing happens with my son.
*Therapist:* Good idea; it would help your son also learn how to moderate irritation at frustrations and disagreements.
*Patient:* Huh.

The patient stayed on the topic and added more information. The therapist helped the patient put each piece of the conversation in sequence and consider who felt what emotion and when. Patient and therapist clarified together that both father and son were angry, and why.

The patient went on to say he regretted how he had spoken angrily to the therapist. He experienced and then told the therapist about emotions related to his embarrassment in that moment with the therapist. He felt he had lapsed in control of his anger in the argument with his son and had been overly harsh in his criticism. The therapist was observing, in this moment, an adaptive level of control over the emergent sense of shame. Also, the patient had learned it was safe to call his feelings "anger."

# Ideational Control Processes

The general goal is to process emotional meanings in a well-modulated state even when the topics are distressing. Some general categories of defensive ideational control processes were observed in the research of independent observers reviewing therapy recordings (Horowitz 1997, 2016a, 2016b; Horowitz et al. 1990, 1993, 1994a, 1994b, 1996b). The maneuvers included altering the immediate topic under joint attention, altering concepts within a topic, altering the time frame under consideration, and altering the focus on appraising realistic or fantastical thinking. These ideational control processes are inferred to organize flow preconsciously, and different outcomes can be reliably observed in the states of mind of the patients in therapy recordings. The generalized theory of processes and outcomes is summarized in Table 4.1.

As noted in Table 4.1, therapy conversations about difficult topics work best when the patient is in a relatively well-modulated state of mind. If the re-schematization stage is reached, attitudinal change can alter preconscious templates for relating self to others. These deeper stages of exploratory psychotherapies are typically aimed at personality growth as well as working through past adverse events.

The aim of this stage of treatment is to help a patient alter schemas of self, another person, and predicted transactions between them. In undermodulated states, dissociation, rage, or separation anxiety may disrupt adaptive processing. In overmodulated states, the therapist may observe defensive maneuvers such as grandiosity or devaluing of another person to protect self-esteem.

Relevant observations of these schematic control processes and their outcomes in different states of mind are shown in Table 4.2.

The therapist can help the patient stabilize their working state, observe their own ideational flow, clarify maladaptive social patterns, and interpret the preconscious schemas that organize those patterns. The patient's attitudes can advance toward a more realistic understanding of the relationship between self and others. The result may be a new capacity for emotionally explicit expression during psychotherapy, and also in conversations with others to resolve relationship disputes and prevent ruptures. That is, the patient may learn from therapy sessions how to calibrate the amount of negative feeling expressed in the actual

**Table 4.1** Ideational control processes observed in different states

| Process of control | State-of-mind outcome | | |
|---|---|---|---|
| | **Overmodulated** | **Well-modulated** | **Undermodulated** |
| **Altering topics of attention** | Does not present stressful topics; instead selects obscuring or misleading alternative topics | Expresses a potentially stressful topic to a degree that can tolerate the evoked emotion | Overwhelming emotions may disorganize thinking |
| **Altering concepts** | Presents an overgeneralized discussion or too quickly switches back and forth | Communicates key facts and emotions | Fragments of sensation and ideas are presented disjointedly |
| **Altering time frame** | Shows disruptive or confusing shifts in temporal frame | Displays a coherent framing of time (past, present, future) or imaginary perspectives | Makes chaotic time references |
| **Altering focus on reality vs. fantasy** | Shows disruptive or confusing shifts between logical reasoning and fantasy | Balances between rational planning and fantasy | Is unable to follow a realistic thread of reasoning |

transactions within close relationships. They can learn how to calm self, negotiate disputes successfully, and preserve constancy with others.

The control processes in Tables 4.1 and 4.2 may be observed in the present moment of a therapy session. Other defense maneuvers may occur over extended periods as part of **character**[1] patterns. If so, it may be helpful to share formulations with the patient about habitually used defense mechanisms. I summarize some of these here.

---

[1] Character: Learned, enduring (but only slowly changing) attitudes and cognitive maps that lend continuity over time to a sense of identity and constancy in attachments.

Table 4.2   Schematic control processes and state observation

| Process of control | State-of-mind outcome | | |
|---|---|---|---|
| | **Overmodulated** | **Well-modulated** | **Undermodulated** |
| **Altering self-schemas** | Expresses excessively grand beliefs about self to ward off shame | Reappraises negative self-appraisals; restores self-esteem | Displays dissociative shifts in self-attribution |
| **Altering schema of other person** | Deflates the internal understanding of other to inflate self-esteem | Shows enriched understanding of others' motives | Expresses excessive rage at other |
| **Altering RRMs** | Reverses roles to augment self-appraisal | Displays sagacious monitoring of others' intentions | Expresses panic at impending separation |

*Note.* RRM, role-relationship model.

**Displacement**[2] occurs when the individual transfers feelings arising toward one person to some other person or object. As an example, when reprimanded by a supervisor at work, a person may tactfully submit to that powerful other, yet go home and kick the family dog or yell at a child for a minor infraction. *Projection* is a related defense. It involves displacing onto the other person a disavowed aspect of the self. For example, a person who is avoiding their own incipient guilt may instead look for some vexing attribute to criticize in another person.

In a variation called **projective identification**,[3] a patient may provoke another person into becoming irritable. If the other reacts, the patient's own reactive anger seems justified as a response to the other person's unfairly hostile behavior. Now the patient avoids shame or guilt at being indignant. Provoking the other person into hostility

[2] Displacement: Shifting a feeling from one person to another object or person.
[3] Projective identification: A complex form of projection in which actions provoke another person to feel that which is projected, such as anger, thus justifying the self in being angry at the other.

provides a basis for attributing blame to someone other than the self. It can be a mechanism employed in passive-aggressive personality styles.

In *reaction formation*, a buried idea or feeling is replaced by an emphasis on its opposite. For example, an older boy who is jealous of a baby brother might harbor a fantasy that if the baby died, he would again be the center of his parents' attention. Having had such a fantasy, he unconsciously realizes that it is "bad." He replaces the wish to be rid of his little brother with an exaggerated concern for the baby's welfare. If his conflict is intense, the reaction formation may lead to problematic symptoms. For instance, the boy might feel a compulsion to check on the baby every 15 minutes throughout the night to make sure he is safe from suffocating.

**Repression**[4] is a complex defense mechanism usually formulated as a buried memory. Emergence needs to be assessed carefully, because true and false fragments can surface from a long repression, such as from childhood trauma.

Suppose a child witnesses a disturbing event (e.g., seeing parents screaming and hitting each other). The child etches such images into a vivid memory. Recollection could be terrifying. That child could pre-consciously plan to avoid all arguments. The unconscious mind acts as if it once recorded this rule: "If you get angry, then you get out of control, and your world will be shattered. So, you must never get angry, and you should ignore frustrations and give in to others. You must keep a lid on any fleck of hostility." As an adult, they might do so. If the plan is not modified by re-schematizing experiences, the patient will be unassertive and emotionally insulated.

As an adult in therapy, such a person is able to develop better schemas for coping. The goal is experiencing, tolerating, and governing anger, because well-modulated irritation can lead to successful changes in relationships.

In therapy, especially in the re-schematization stage, a patient who has habitually and defensively avoided disputes or self-assertion of any kind can learn that frustration can be expressed safely rather than in a dreaded out-of-control state. They can practice successful negotiation to meet one's own needs. No one has to get physically hurt; firm assertiveness that emphasizes collaboration and cooperation within personal limits will suffice. Usefully expressed, a tactful and even

---

[4] Repression: A defensive maneuver in which memories and fantasies are unconsciously represented but inhibited from emerging consciously.

**Table 4.3**   Obstacles to therapy with people who habitually inhibit ideas

| Defensive style | Therapeutic technique |
| --- | --- |
| Global or selective inattention with impressionistic rather than accurate discourse about situations | Encourage talk and provide plausible verbal representations for ideas and feelings. |
| Limited disclosure; inhibitions of ideas | Ask for details, and then construct cause-and-effect sequences. |
| Short-circuit to erroneous conclusions | Keep the topic open, slow down, and emphasize step-by-step decision-making. |
| Misinterpretations based on stereotypes | Interpret what is realistically likely; differentiate that from what is most dreaded and what is ideally desired. Clarify time frames, distinguishing past from possible future. |

slightly hostile message tells others to desist in unacceptable or abusive behavior. Values shift from "anger is always bad" to "anger can be adaptive or maladaptive depending on the way it is expressed."

# Emotional Expressions Dislocated From Ideas Involved in Activating Affect

Some patients have a style that involves expressing feelings internally but lacking words for clearly identifying those emotions or why they occurred. They habitually inhibit some relevant ideas. They experience memories as sensory impressions without rational appraisal of sequences. These styles can be counteracted by techniques shown in Table 4.3.

One of the most common habitual defenses observed by therapists is **intellectualization**.[5] The patient avoids expressing feelings with

---

[5] Intellectualization: A defensive maneuver in which emotions are not represented in talk or thought, although related ideas may be put into words.

**Table 4.4**  Obstacles to therapy with people who habitually avoid emotion

| Defensive style | Therapeutic technique |
| --- | --- |
| Has an excessively detailed but peripheral approach to talking about situations | Ask for personalized meanings. |
| Avoids disclosure of emotion | Interpret linkage of emotional meanings to ideational meanings; ask about bodily sensations. |
| Juggles opposing sets of meanings back and forth | Hold discussions on one valence of a topic; interpret defensive shifting and the meanings it conceals. |
| Endlessly ruminates without reaching decisions about how to act | Interpret reasons for warding off reaching decisions and for impulsive actions rather than carefully chosen ones. |

rigid generalizations. The topic brought forth in therapy may be potentially emotional, but the patient treats the concepts as if they were in a public sphere rather than in their own mind. The typical observations and the potentially useful techniques in the moment are summarized in Table 4.4.

# Patients Who Distort Reality for Self-Enhancement

Some patients shift blame for losses and traumas to external factors or people. They distort reality to protect the self from shame. This is a characteristic of a narcissistic personality style, which will be discussed more in Chapter 7 ("Managing Narcissistic Traits"); some techniques are summarized in Table 4.5.

# Summary

Adverse childhood events predispose some people to disturbances in emotional regulation, leading to both underregulated and overmodulated states of mind (Lieberman 2008). The therapist's personalized

Table 4.5   Obstacles to therapy with people who distort reality for self-enhancement

| Defensive style | Therapeutic technique |
| --- | --- |
| Focuses on praise and blame issues; is deceitful | Avoid being provoked into either praising or blaming; do not accuse of lying. |
| Avoids or disavows information that deflates self-esteem | Use tactful timing and wording to counteract denials and deceits. |
| Alters meanings about who did what to whom—that is, exaggerates the importance of what the other person did to blame them for what the self minimized to reduce self-criticism | Consistently redefine meanings and encourage realistic appraisals while bolstering against shame. |
| Pays excessive attention to self-enhancement | Cautiously deflate grandiose meanings while empathetically emphasizing realistic skills and capacities. |
| Dislocates bad attributes of self to others | Clarify who is who in terms of acts, intentions, and expectations. |
| Forgives self too easily when some remorse is realistically justified; denies any culpability | Support self-esteem with a genuine interest in the patient while working toward an appropriate sense of responsibility; help plan for realistic acts of remorse without excessive shame. |

techniques aim to provide enough safety to promote working states of mind during a session. Undercontrolled emotion can lead to shifts into states too flooded with feelings to process ideas in a re-narrative mode. Emotions that are too rigidly controlled lead to overmodulated states of mind. The therapist helps the patient safely contain and express feelings while reasoning together about meanings in well-modulated states. This may include tactics to counteract defenses and create a dose-by-dose, slowed-down processing of reasons that negative emotions have been intensified.

The felt presence of safety in dialogue with a therapist may enable a patient to calibrate emotional intensity, which helps a patient 1) pay attention, 2) increase self-reflective awareness, 3) reappraise beliefs and develop insight, 4) accept negative feelings, and 5) develop plans for better interpersonal transactions.

# Key Points

- Defensiveness can be counteracted without having to interpret the defense.
- Defensive obstacles are best addressed by helping the patient stabilize well-modulated working states during therapy sessions and beyond.
- Interpreting a habitual defensive style may be valuable in a deeper stage of therapy, when origins may be explored.
- In deeper work, a configuration of desired, dreaded, and defensive factors for a particular theme and pattern can be clarified.
- Slowing down and parsing reactions in a conversational style advances the processing and integration of a stressor topic. In this way, past traumatic memories can be reorganized in multiple registries of preserved memories, fantasies, and attitudes.

# 5

# Paying Attention to the Patient's Current Level of Personality Functioning

Formulating individualized personality patterns helps a clinician understand the patient's capacity to use the learning opportunities of therapy sessions (Shedler and Westen 2007). Patients with lower cognitive capacity may be slower in learning new attitudes and need more therapy than patients at high levels of functioning. Techniques for increasing emotional control and augmenting thought processes for realistic processing of relationship scenarios can promote growth, even in patients with only insecure assumptions of constancy in connections with others.

Impoverishment of executive control functions is hard to formulate but important to observe—the repetitive maladaptive patterns are complex and variable. Patients at lower levels of personality functioning may have dissociations between states of mind. Sometimes very different preconscious schemas of self and other dominate the organization of beliefs within the pattern. Sudden changes of emotion (e.g., from demanding affectionate attention to blaming the other for abandonment) may occur. Some paranoid beliefs may emerge in one state and not be recognized as of the self in a dissociated other state.

Different attitudes about self (e.g., self-worth, accuracy of self-view, self-direction) may prevail in alternative experiences and social behaviors. In addition, lower levels of emotional control capacity may interfere with affective tolerance. Intense feelings of anger, guilt, shame, and despair may lead to cognitive disorganization or irrational transference reactions.

During conversations with the therapist, some patients may have diminished capacity for understanding the therapist. If the therapist offers long interpretations, as in how childhood attitudes manifest in current interpersonal patterns, the patient may be unable to follow the reasoning. The therapist should parse their remarks into smaller amounts of information for the patient to process in the present moment (Horowitz 2019; Lindfors et al. 2014; Mullin and Hilsenroth 2014).

Personality disorders and ways of formulating disturbed traits of social behavior are still a debated topic in psychoanalytic theory, psychological testing, and contemporary classification efforts. Classifications of personality disorders in DSM-5 (American Psychiatric Association 2013, 2022) differ from those in earlier DSM editions. An alternative model suggested by a committee of psychologists and psychiatrists but rejected by the board of trustees, "Alternative DSM-5 Model for Personality Disorders," is included in Section III, "Emerging Measures and Models" (p. 761 of DSM-5; p. 881 of DSM-5-TR).

Meanwhile, multiple personality disorder diagnoses were omitted from ICD-11 (World Health Organization 2022). Descriptions of traits and capacities were included. A process of changing descriptors is very much in the spirit of these times—people are complicated and do not fit well into a single class. But clinically, levels of disturbance are important in formulating the patient's present capacity for adaptive maintenance of self-esteem and effective social behavior. A simplified approach to classification is offered here.

# Level of Personality Functioning

Research has indicated the importance of identity, relationship affiliations, and control of emotional behavior in self-appraisals and approaches to social connections. The American Psychiatric Association's diagnostic revision committees developed a framework for assessing these important social cognition variables in a range of ratings from 0 (high-level functioning) to 4 (very disturbed) (see Table 2, "Level of Personality Functioning Scale," DSM-5-TR, American Psychiatric Association 2022, p. 895) (Bender et al. 2011; Skodol et al.

2011). These dimensional and transdiagnostic ratings drew from research into the quantitative rating of social cognitive schematization as a dispositional variable that has been demonstrated to predict differential symptom outcomes as correlated to various actions by a therapist in the process of treatments (Diener and Monroe 2011; Gamache et al. 2009; Høglend et al. 2006; Horowitz et al. 1984; Mullin and Hilsenroth 2014; Piper et al. 1991).

Many investigators favor a dimensional approach (Vanheule 2012; Westen et al. 2012; Widiger 2011) to clarify commonalities in technique for a given typology (Lingiardi and McWilliams 2017). Some scales have shown promise for qualitative assessment of such traitlike dimensions in the social cognition of psychiatric patients. Of these, the most relevant measure is the Object Relations Inventory (Blatt and Luyten 2009; Blatt et al. 1997), which yields a subscale representing the observer's inference of a subject's current level of self-other differentiation. As used by Bers et al. (2013), the subscale has 10 levels, from low (lack of differentiation of persons) to high (reflectively constructed and integrated representation of self and relationships).

The issues of dissociative self-states and lapses in emotional regulation have been discussed in many ways in relation to trauma and adverse childhood experiences. With a group at the University of California San Francisco, I conducted research on brief psychotherapy for stress response syndromes, studying disposition interacting with therapist action, patient alliance experiences, and symptomatic outcomes. After finding adequate reliability of clinician ratings, we used the range of scores on the Organizational Levels of Self-Other Schematization (OLSOS) as a dispositional variable to examine how specific techniques in the psychotherapy process led to outcomes assessed on symptomatic results in posttreatment evaluations. OLSOS ratings predicted better results for supportive techniques in therapy of patients who were more disturbed in social cognitive capacities and better results for interpreting and emotionally evocative techniques in persons with more self-coherence, relationship capacity, and self-control of emotional states (Horowitz 2014, 2016a; Horowitz et al. 1984). The OLSOS categories are summarized in Table 5.1.

The levels of functioning in Table 5.1 are harmonious, conflicted, vulnerable, very disturbed, and fragmented. "No observed patterns of disturbance" means that the person displays *harmonious* (formerly called "healthy") qualities, such as coherence of sense of self over time. The *conflicted* level was formerly called "neurotic"; *vulnerable* was "narcissistic"; *very disturbed* was "borderline"; and *fragmented* was

**Table 5.1** Organizational levels of self-other schematization

| | |
|---|---|
| Harmonious | • Maintains a shared understanding of the present context with significant others.<br>- Exhibits state transitions appropriate to situations.<br>- Examines realistic pros and cons to reach rational choices of action.<br>- Is grounded in self and views others as separate people with their own intentions and expectations.<br>• Has perspectives on relationships that approximate social norms.<br>• Displays positive and negative valences in meaningful relationships that are integrated, allowing a sense of constancy.<br>• Possesses emotional governance that prevents out-of-control states from rupturing relationships. |
| Conflicted | • Displays alternative states based on fluctuating attitudes about a relationship.<br>• Exhibits state transitions that occur between positive and negative moods, but memories of each state are remembered rather than dissociated.<br>• Demonstrates fears of rejection that limit attachments to others or fears of subordination that limit cooperation.<br>• Appraises self with a variety of critical judgments, some too harsh and some too lax. |
| Vulnerable | • Has excessive intensity or significant flattening of affect and tone, to a degree outside of cultural norms.<br>• Shows surprising shifts from vigor and boldness to apathy or impulsivity.<br>• Seems to have an idiosyncratic perceptual experience of the world.<br>• Has a sense of self-regard that deteriorates under stress, criticism, and increased pressure to perform.<br>• Uses grandiose supports of self-esteem to protect from feelings of inferiority or enfeeblement.<br>• Erupts in undermodulated rage at others who are perceived as insulting or blamed for embarrassment. |

---

**Table 5.1** Organizational levels of self-other schematization (*continued*)

| | |
|---|---|
| Very Disturbed | • Commits major errors in self-other attribution.<br>• Exhibits explosive state transitions.<br>• Projects undesirable self-attributes and emotions from self to other. The actions of self may be dissociated in memory in terms of who did or felt what, and shifts in self-state may be accompanied by dissociations of memory of what happened in the alternative state of mind.<br>• In memories, confusingly combines fantasy with reality.<br>• Exhibits alternative personalities. |
| Fragmented | • Becomes chaotically distracted and even psychotic.<br>• Shows affect and tone that either vary in a labile fashion or are overly restricted to one state, with an intensity level (high or low) that is well outside of cultural norms.<br>• Displays massive chaos of selfhood; frequently feels as if under attack and may attack others seen as predators.<br>• Withdraws in a self-protecting coping effort that, to others, appears bizarre. |

---

"psychotic." The dimensional model of Table 5.1 is less complex than the Alternative DSM-5 Model for Personality Disorders described earlier in this chapter (American Psychiatric Association 2022).

Personality traits such as self-abasement may cross these dimensions. Suppose a clinician conducts therapy with a patient who has an excessively dependent pattern. The patient desires to be taken care of and fears that their wish will be frustrated because they are not interesting enough for others to pay attention to their needs. If functioning at a *conflicted* level, the patient may say, in effect, "I need care, and sometimes I get it. I show my appreciation and so gratify my providers. When no one is available, I feel distressed but do not abuse substances because I expect help soon." In contrast, if at a *vulnerable* level, the patient may say, in effect, "I need care but am afraid to ask for it. People dislike a dependent person unless they can take advantage of them and then leave them on the roadside. So I pretend to be independent and conceal my yearning for guidance and support by drinking." Functioning at a *very disturbed* level, the patient might say, in effect, "People should know I need help without me saying anything. Some people persecute and neglect me. They ought to be punished for not caring for me." Details about therapy techniques for each level are described in Table 5.2.

# Personality Development

A patient's unharmonized level of personality functioning as currently instantiated may be a regression from a higher level of developmental achievement (due to a factor such as stress), or it may be the highest level of personality functioning this patient has achieved. If the lower level of functioning is habitual, then the clinician must address personality structure as part of the re-schematization stage of therapy. Insecure, anxious, and avoidant attachment patterns in the vulnerable levels may be due to adverse childhood events that led to developmental traumas or neglect. In addition, genetics and biological damage can affect the complex transactions between biological, psychological, and social factors.

## Biopsychosocial Interactions

Vulnerability in brain circuitry for social behaviors can limit a patient's capacity for social attachment behaviors. The circuitries involve the salience network of important cortical and subcortical anatomical regions of the brain. These may affect partnering; in a previously connected adult, damage may lead to loss of capacity—Alzheimer's disease is one example. Prior bonding patterns may not be maintained, and both partners may experience reduced rewards from social experiences. Psychological responses such as depressive and suicidal states may result. The partner may view the altered patterns in the person with dementia as a "personality change."

## Psychological Factors in Development

Sigmund Freud believed that some people fixate on an early stage of child development rather than continuing to learn capacities with advancing age. Erik Erikson went beyond that idea of early childhood fixations to a model of adaptive change over a life cycle, from infancy to old age. A patient might stall rather than advance in that model, and formulating developmental arrests may help the clinician consider techniques for helping the patient resume growth.

**Table 5.2**  Technique related to current level of functioning

| Level | Technique |
| --- | --- |
| Conflicted and vulnerable | The patient may develop transference feelings leading to sessions containing emotionally intense states, but these feelings are usually tolerable if contained within a good therapeutic alliance. When the patient shifts into a state with negative transference feelings, the therapist contrasts these with the already experienced and realistic frame of the alliance. Then clarifications and interpretations may be processed and attitudes changed. |
| Very disturbed and fragmented | The patient may lack a basic sense of security in a relationship, and that may manifest as a variety of distancing, distrusting, or provocative behaviors. In some states, they lose realistic perceptual appraisals of the therapeutic alliance. They may experience the therapist's effort at clarification of a dysfunctional belief as if the therapist were attacking or insulting. Then negative transference feelings occur. |
| | Techniques should not be overly interpretive but rather focus on repairing the sense of rupture in a caring, empathetic relationship between patient and therapist. Short, empathetic statements by the therapist may help. These repair techniques usually need multiple repetitions for the patient to learn new schemas. It may be helpful to pair insight-promoting clarifications with statements that are positive and hopeful. For example, "I think you are expressing your irritation at me in a useful way. It can further my understanding of what's on your mind." |

For these reasons, a social developmental theory can lead to individualized inferences of what might be a next developmental aim (Horowitz 2016a; McWilliams 2011). Here we consider only a rough general format. Table 5.3 shows common developmental milestones for the factors we have been discussing: identity, relationships, and emotional control.

Sharing ideas about development with a patient can provide a way forward. Psychoeducation goes both ways: the patient clarifies their own cultural developments and conflicts, and the therapist helps in providing understanding from science and their own experience. The

**Table 5.3   Developmental map**

| Period | Social expectations | Identity | Relationships | Emotional control |
|---|---|---|---|---|
| Infancy | Achieve attunement; learn to walk and talk | Formulate first beliefs about the bodily self | Develop first understanding of self as attached to others (vs. insecurity) | Acquire trust and hope (vs. terror) |
| Early childhood | Increase bodily control; develop sense of right and wrong; learn communication skills | Acquire sense of competence of self (vs. identity disturbance) | Become familiar with roles for social interactions (vs. deficits in social cognition) | Begin confident exploration and learn how to recover from frustration (vs. fearful avoidance or tantrums) |
| Middle childhood | Relate to peers; form close friendships; learn to work on one's own; enlarge moral sense | Form multiple self-schemas and flexibly shift between them (vs. self-doubt) | Find multiple RRMs of friendship (vs. chronic loneliness) | Follow the rules of social context (vs. impulsive patterns) |
| Early adolescence | Accept one's changing body; experiment with sexuality; forge peer groups; develop work and recreational abilities | Resiliently use multiple self-schemas (vs. dissociation) | Try out alternative roles and scripts for sexuality, disputes, and commitments with adaptive learning (vs. projective distortions) | Make apt value choices (vs. excessive isolation or conformity) |

**Table 5.3 Developmental map** (*continued*)

| Period | Social expectations | Identity | Relationships | Emotional control |
|--------|--------------------|----------|---------------|-------------------|
| Late adolescence | Extend understanding of gender and sexual roles; develop specific skills for work and socialization; learn to balance cooperation, competition, and independence | Form complex self-schemas (vs. alternative dissociated selves) | Try out and learn cooperative and competitive RRMs (vs. withdrawal or attack) | Improve self-modulation of emotion (vs. disturbed and dysphoric moods) |
| Young adulthood | Relate to social systems of work, families, and communities | Form harmonious configurations of self-schemas (vs. conflictual configurations) | Find harmonious supraordinate configurations of RRMs (vs. isolation and purposelessness) | Regulate mood transitions (vs. explosive mood shifts or anhedonia) |
| Middle adulthood | Share values and power; transmit skills to younger people | Conduct realistic self-appraisal and acceptance (vs. self-disgust) | Achieve relationship complexity schemas (vs. conflictual dissociations) | Appropriately use power (vs. unrestrained self-aggrandizement or giving up) |
| Late adulthood | Accept aging body; confront transience; convey wisdom | Wisely re-narrate self-organization (vs. terror or bitterness) | Develop schemas of the future in which valued relationships survive personal death | Gain flexibility in relinquishing control |

*Note.* RRM, role-relationship model.

goal is to understand maladaptive attitudes and deficits and learn new ways to deactivate those that have become entrenched.

The therapist also helps the patient think in ways that amount to a re-narration of specific family and community memories and histories. That process includes explicating conflicts in what the patient once believed they ought to become and clarifying new goals for the future. A review of the theory of development can help, as summarized in Table 5.3.

In considering individualized developmental narratives, therapists should clarify differences between their own cultural background and that of the patient. Identifying shared and different backgrounds for goals, values, and purpose can be a valuable technique, because patients can sense those of the therapist but may also misinterpret them.

To reduce the activity of older cognitive schemas, the patient can learn newer, more adaptive ones. The old ones are not erased—some patients expect erasure, but that does not happen. What does happen is less-frequent intrusive flashbacks and fantasies of childhood adversities and more tolerance of stressful situations that in the past would have triggered fear, anger, or withdrawal.

In other words, the complex associational linkages may still lead to predictive coding for expected or intended relationship patterns when emotional triggers occur. The patient may enter an adaptive or maladaptive state depending on whether the adult-learned schemas are the active organizers, dominant over the older schemas, which are probably from childhood relationships.

Conversations that are psychoeducative about this aspect of personality psychology may help patients enhance the very important capacity of reflective self-awareness, which could also be called adaptive mindfulness. Such conversations can improve the therapeutic alliance even if the patient is much older than the therapist. A young therapist can reassure an older patient that although they have not lived to the patient's place in a life cycle, they have learned in training how to understand these issues. Therapists also learn about life from the experiences understood together with their patients.

The summary provided in the map of development over a generalized life cycle can help a therapist clarify emotions from social stressors. For example, in middle adulthood, a patient may feel depressed and irritable about a social situation in which power differentials and identity politics need to be clarified.

As an illustration, consider the case of a 40-year-old social worker who was diagnosed with major depressive disorder in interviews with his primary care internist. He refused his physician's recommendation of antidepressant medications and was referred to a therapy-oriented clinician. When the new therapist asked about his current situation, he reported a recent divorce, meager income, and feeling stuck in his job in a disrupted economy. He shifted into tears when the therapist summarized what they had heard so far. This crying state seemed to occur when he experienced understanding in the form of a warm, accepting restatement of how he felt powerless in many sectors.

*Therapist:* Now that we have reviewed your history, I think we might note that you sometimes have states of mind that are marked with a sense of low self-worth. I heard you speak of helping others in your workplace. Do they find that of value?

*Patient:* I don't make as much money as some of them.

*Therapist:* I wonder if that is balanced by being of help?

*Patient:* I just feel I am not amounting to much.

*Therapist:* I know you got a divorce a couple of years ago, but I am impressed that you and your former partner are still friends. That shows something good, doesn't it?

The therapist was assessing this patient as able to function at a conflicted (higher) level of personality functioning. Thus they asked questions that might derail a patient operating at a lower level. The patient indicated this higher level of functioning with the adaptive way in which he ended the session.

*Patient:* I know from your clock we are ending soon, but I kind of want to think about that further in our next session.

*Therapist:* And then we can talk about what you think about this when you review this session in your mind before our next time together.

The therapist is using a tactful "homework assignment" without going into detail. They are also thinking about topics such as possible futures and goals that might be gradually considered. Meanwhile, the therapist plans to emphasize that the patient can continue taking care of his well-being through good levels of exercise, sleep, nutrition, and self-presentation.

Damage from adverse childhood events and attachment deficits can contribute to poor current social abilities. A patient may try to engage others in a preliminary relationship using maneuvers that repel rather than attract. New learning can take place in the increasingly secure therapeutic alliance. This process is usually slow. Small encounters can teach new ways, verbal and nonverbal, as in the following example.

> Seymour is a 28-year-old patient who operates at a vulnerable level of personality functioning. He had reported in earlier therapy sessions how he had occasional depressive states of social withdrawal, with easily triggered anxious and lonely states of mind. In some therapy sessions, Seymour shared a sense of connection with the therapist, appreciating empathetic comments and clarifications. At times, the clinician observed a shift in conversation pattern from direct verbal and nonverbal messages on a shared topic to a state of disconnection.
>
> Of note, the clinician observed moments of spasmodic smiling with coquettish head movements. This interrupted a calmer stance of eye contact and appropriate sequences of verbal messages. In the course of formulating, the therapist explored the concept that this was a defensive gambit when disconnected, an attempt to avoid loss of relationship using a chronic maladaptive pattern related to a normal adaptive pattern for first social engagements. The patient was coping with their disconnection by nonverbally saying in effect, "I am a nice attractive person." In therapy, this behavior served as a defensive maneuver, avoiding possible shame in the flow of self-descriptive talk.
>
> The therapist then observed that when they talked slowly and repeated what had just been discussed, Seymour's avoidance of facial messaging was reduced, protecting him from embarrassment over the messages he had been giving before the fake-seeming smiling behavior. The patient appeared to listen and, when talking next, returned to reporting an awkward, embarrassing exchange with a coworker he wished to befriend. The safety of the therapeutic alliance seemed to have made this possible.

In a subsequent session, the therapist tried to clarify further:

*Therapist:* I notice that you sometimes want to get off a topic that I try to keep in our discussion and that you use some facial expressions that may not have the effect you want on other people.
*Patient:* Can you show me what I do?
*Therapist:* I think so. First, let me set the stage. I am pretending to be you. In my mind I want to say we are okay with each other, and I am not trying to evade you.
*Patient:* Got it, pretend away.

*Therapist:* Then this [gives a fake smile with rapid nodding]. You might slow that down; if I'm right, it could work better [repeats smile slowly].

*Patient:* I feel a little embarrassed. But maybe I can learn something [practices a more genuine smile].

*Therapist:* Yes, that works, I think.

This example is the first step in a shared understanding of an entrenched pattern that functions preconsciously and was not consciously decided on in the past. In the safety of the therapeutic alliance, a momentary rupture due to anticipated shame with a defensive cover was inferred by the therapist. They intended in their remarks to protect Seymour from his preconsciously predicted embarrassment. They framed remarks and role-played in the hope of helping the patient express a stressful recent memory with tolerance for its embarrassing innuendos. The experience of protection from a searing emotion helped build a new relationship schema, with more trust in how another might stay tuned to expression of negative feelings.

This example relates to a task noted for young adults in Table 5.3, learning more about how to regulate smoother mood transitions (vs. explosive mood shifts or anhedonia).

## Summary

A patient's current level of functioning may change with new stressors and associational triggers to traumatic memories. The emotional intensity may disorganize thinking and emotional control even more than is customary. Metabolic changes may also alter executive functioning, emotional control, and a patient's capacity for realistically understanding immediate social situations. Observation is important and can lead to formulating levels of development in schemas of self and others, as well as apt social transactional sequences.

## Key Points

- Formulating individualized personality patterns helps a clinician understand the patient's capacity to use the learning opportunities of therapy sessions.
- In patients with lower functioning, the most important on-the-spot technical implications involve attention to the repair of ruptures in the therapeutic alliance. This can be achieved by slow,

small-dose repetitions of emotional signals, verbally and non-verbally, and clarification of the therapist's intentions in making remarks.

- A young therapist can reassure an older patient that although they have not lived to the patient's place in a life cycle, they have learned in training how to understand these issues.
- Therapists can gradually form a shared understanding with patients of an entrenched pattern that previously functioned only preconsciously. Thus it can be examined in conscious self-reflections, and new attitudes can be formed to replace it.
- Practice in relationships helps new schemas to evolve even further than in therapy sessions.

# 6

# Correcting Schemas From Experiences in a Therapeutic Alliance

A s a patient learns from experiences in an enriching therapeutic alliance, new attachment relationship schemas can develop. Instead of preconsciously expecting coldness or exploitation, a connection of trust is codified. The previous patterns from insecure, anxious, or avoidant models of attachment in close relationships may emerge as transference feelings or resistances, but the real safety, compassion, empathy, and constancy of therapy interactions can modify those expectations.

Transference feelings may be expressed verbally or nonverbally; the therapist clarifies and interprets by talking about how this is to be understood and processed within the boundaries of respective roles and expected transactions in the therapy framework. This new learning of self-other intentions and engagement possibilities is an aspect of re-schematization.

Freud (1915) noted how a learning experience occurred when the therapist did not 1) coldly rebuff the patient's expression of positive transference messages or 2) engage romantically. This technique of understanding, acceptance, clarification, and interpretation has since been confirmed as valuable (Blatman 2015). Responsive, positive countertransference impulses are to be recognized and contained within the therapist's mind.

Negative transference and countertransference tendencies are also contained as times for clarification and interpretation of the realities of the actual therapeutic framework. Negative moments of reacting in therapy are more common in patients with childhood experiences such as abuse; to see if repetitions of such episodes might recur, they may challenge the therapist (Briere and Elliot 2003).

A patient may use flirtatious behavior as an unconsciously motivated test to see if the therapist will be a strong, caring figure who remains within a professional frame. Although the patient may appear to be asking for erotic attention, in such scenarios, the patient may not unconsciously want a sexual encounter; instead, they have an unconscious aim to find a figure who can resist sexual impulse and who instead practices appropriate compassion without crossing boundaries. The following case example shows how proper technique can lead to new learning of adult schemas for attachment in such situations.

Amber, a 34-year-old health professional, met diagnostic criteria for major depressive disorder. Her initial symptoms had been ameliorated with support and motivational techniques to counteract her excessive solitude, which limited life quality for relationships. In the re-schematization stage of her treatment, she was exploring deeper patterns of seemingly inevitable intimate relationship disputes and losses. In romantic opportunities, she tended to repeat a maladaptive pattern. A sequence began impulsively in a state of loneliness, leading to an imperative search for someone to appease her longing to be loved. Without attention of that sort, she felt fragile and at times almost without a sense of identity.

She would quickly fall in love with anyone who showed interest in her. All too soon, she felt sexually used, deserted, and angry. The desperate loneliness that followed would restart the cycle, as she impulsively latched on to any next partner. Then she gave up in favor of depressed solitude. When that was intolerable, the cycle was again repeated.

With her therapist, Amber reviewed memories related to the pattern. Her uncle sexually assaulted her when she was 15 years old. At the time of the abuse, she did not feel mistreated and distressed; rather, she felt that the sexual encounter was a consensual one of romantic true love and shared erotic pleasure. Their relationship was concealed from family and friends. Yet, 2 years later, at the age of 17, she came to view this episode in retrospect as a betrayal of her trust. From that time on, she carried a grievance against her uncle.

She recognized that she had repeatedly reenacted unsatisfying sexual relationships with men. She felt pessimistic about the future,

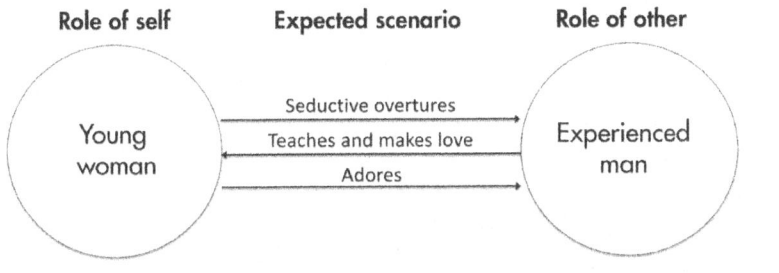

**Figure 6.1** Early phase of Amber's maladaptive pattern.

predicting for herself a "life of sorrows" instead of a "happy life," which she defined as marriage and children. It was not enough that she was successful and secure in her profession.

At the end of a session, she told her therapist she loved him. She stood up and offered her open arms and body for a hug. She seemed to be in an altered state of mind organized by the relationship model diagrammed in Figure 6.1. The therapist did not reciprocate the roles depicted and instead asked her to sit down so that they could talk this over.

Amber sat down looking distressed. The therapist said calmly, "You look embarrassed. Please don't be. I want to talk this situation over with you, without hugging." Amber then cried and expressed feelings of being rejected, shimmering in and out of an undermodulated state. She then shifted back into a well-modulated working state, in which she understood what was going on and could process ideas in conversation. Her memories related to this episode were reappraised and renarrated in subsequent sessions.

In those sessions, the therapist and Amber used verbal labels to clarify the respective roles of self and other as they were enacted in stories about her important previous sexual relationships. Through these discussions, her hopes were clarified and interpreted in relation to the new narratives of her past experiences. The desired role-relationship model (RRM) depicted in Figure 6.1 was clarified, including her usual maladaptive transformation into the dreaded pattern of rejection and desperate loneliness. The end story of the pattern of relationship ruptures is depicted in Figure 6.2.

Therapy dialogues led to progress in further clarifying the realistic roles in their therapeutic alliance. Her trust gradually increased with the therapist's continued noncritical clarifications and interpretations

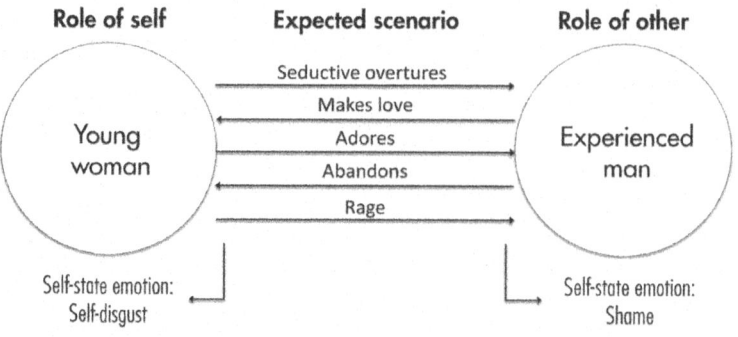

**Figure 6.2   Later phase of Amber's maladaptive pattern.**

that promoted insight. She expressed a braid of emotions and clarified strands of shame, guilt, longing, and bitterness. Above all, she came to express anger and sadness verbally as she reconsidered her adolescent sexual abuse and some exploitative lovers in her recent past.

The consistency and enriched realization of the therapeutic alliance was an important corrective relationship experience. In the new relationship experience, the therapist showed their value of caring for her as a person and their shared interest in promoting her adult personality growth. The frame was clear: a therapeutic alliance as in Figure 6.3.

Figure 6.4 shows the new RRM of the therapeutic alliance as eventually experienced by Amber.

Figures 6.1 to 6.4 follow the same format for noting inferred schemas that probably exist in the patient's repertoire of predictive coding. As already discussed, these types of schemas are called *role-relationship models* (RRMs). They include person attributes (roles) and predictive scenarios—transactive models that are scripts of relationship intentions and expectations. As a part of formulating and sharing insights, a therapist could sketch out RRMs with a patient. For most patients, however, the therapist's technique will involve statements separated by feedback from the patient on how they understood what was just said. To summarize such a technique, examples of the therapist's intended actions and statements to Amber are illustrated in Table 6.1.

For a therapist to enable a patient to learn from new experiences, they need to be aware of and avoid two potential technical errors. That is, the therapist should not be so warm as to indicate a boundary is being crossed, and the therapist should not be so cold as to appear remote, which can be misinterpreted by the patient as rejection. In

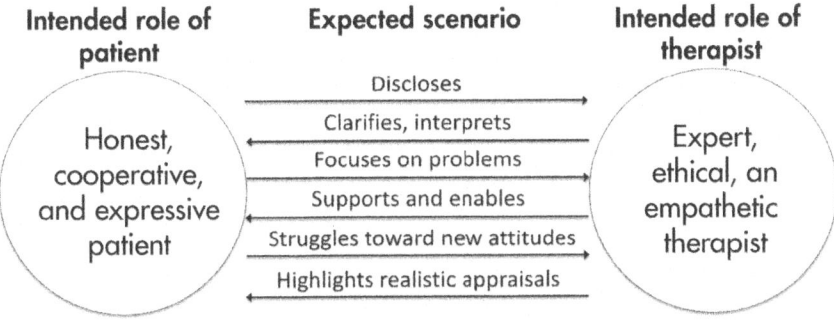

**Figure 6.3    Roles of a relationship in a therapeutic alliance.**

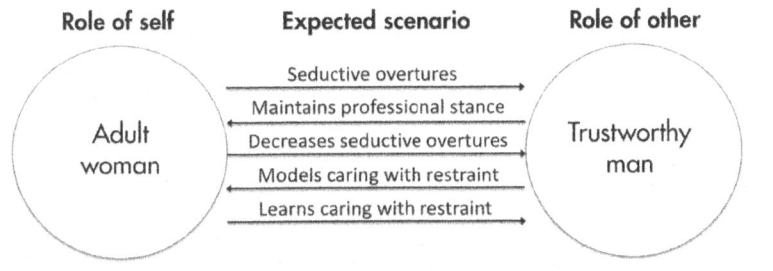

**Figure 6.4    Learning from the evolving therapeutic alliance.**

Amber's case, the therapist maintained eye contact and a calm, friendly facial expression to avoid appearing remote.

As with Amber, a therapist may respond to transference behaviors by defining professional boundaries and emphasizing trust-building and verbal communication. If they feel rejected, the patient may react angrily at first. However, they will eventually recognize that what is occurring in therapy is not rejection—instead, it is a compassionate and restrained form of continuous caring in the safety of a therapeutic alliance, as shown in Figure 6.4.

Amber's case example represents formulations about the therapeutic change made possible by maintaining a therapeutic alliance with a patient who is at a medium-high level of personality functioning. Such progress may be difficult or even impossible with a patient at a low level of personality functioning (Horowitz 2013). For them, such inferences about schemas are too complex to discuss, except piece by piece with repetitions and feedback.

**Table 6.1**  Therapeutic actions

| Action | Sample statement |
| --- | --- |
| Expressing empathy | I understand from what you are saying that you are feeling angry at me because you want us to express affection for one another. |
| Clarifying the framework of therapeutic alliance | You want us to express physical affection for one another, but I cannot reciprocate. |
| Interpreting the transference | Because I decline to hug, I think that you mistakenly experience me as coldly rejecting your feelings. |
| Interpreting the therapeutic alliance | On the contrary, I accept your feelings and am trying to help you understand them. I am acting on your behalf. |
| Clarifying professional boundaries | My job is being your therapist and helping you safely tell me your thoughts and feelings. |
| Expressing noncritical positive regard | My aim is to help you stop repeating a cycle that leads to states of blame, anger, sadness, and self-disgust. |
| Interpreting the therapeutic alliance and contrasting the interpretation of transference | I am not coldly rejecting you, although I know you feel like that's what's happening. |
| Expressing shared values for therapy | I care about your future. |
| Teaching governance of impulses | I hope you can learn to love others in the future by using restraint until it is safe for you to be fully spontaneous. |
| Summarizing new relationship scenario | Increasing your capacities for tolerating this pain can bring you to a state of readiness to both love and be loved with commitment, rather than having a short romance that ends in grievance and feelings of self-disgust. |
| Negotiating and reaffirming therapeutic goals | I am asking you to fully express to me your feelings and to regard restraint as a commitment to honor opportunities that you can make possible in your future. |

DeMasi (2012) puts it succinctly in his review article, one with excellent clinical examples, as the difference between patients who harbor erotic delusions at fragmented levels and patients like Amber who may have states with a *dreamy* rather than *delusional* fantasy of reenactment. For attitudes to change in the direction of new relationships and self-schemas, the patient must have developed capacities for rational understanding of transactions and motives.

## Summary

In the re-schematization stage of therapy, the patient's memories, fantasies, and imagined future can be deeply explored, clarified, and interpreted. Transference feelings are contained and changed in the framework of a constantly developing therapeutic alliance.

## Key Points

- Insecure, anxious, or avoidant models of attachment in close relationships may emerge as transference feelings or resistances, but the real safety, compassion, empathy, and constancy of therapy interactions can modify those expectations.
- Negative moments of reacting in therapy are more common in patients with negative childhood experiences such as abuse, and the patient may challenge the therapist to see whether repetitions of such episodes might recur.
- A therapist should not be so warm as to indicate a boundary crossing; the therapist should not be so cold as to appear remote.
- Role-relationship models are useful tools for formulating because they include both person attributes (roles) and predictive scenarios, which are scripts of relationship intentions and expectations.

# 7

# Managing Narcissistic Traits

Identity disturbances and interpersonal dysfunction are prominent and hard to change in those with narcissistic traits (Diamond et al. 2022; Horowitz 2009; Kernberg 2009). Although high intelligence may be present, these patients may have low self-reflective capacity. Efforts at interpretation may succeed, but they may also lead to identity difficulties and withdrawal due to shame avoidance (Fonagy et al. 2005).

Clinicians experience special challenges when treating patients with narcissistic traits. They may intuitively assess the patient as selfish, grandiose, and callous—hard to like—and find it difficult to muster the compassion needed for an enriched therapeutic alliance. In this chapter, I help the clinician formulate any countertransferences, defensive obstacles, and transferences that such patients may present. It helps to assess whether the patient shows any phenomena of grandiosity that compensate for a warded-off sense of insecurity and impaired self-worth. Recognizing such layers of schemas will help the patient develop relevant techniques to form better relationship patterns and develop realistic goals for self-esteem.

## Narcissistic Traits

A person with narcissistic traits overly attends to sources of power, praise, and embarrassment in the interpersonal field (Horowitz 1981,

2009, 2014, 2018; Kernberg 2009; Kohut 1972, 1977). They try to avoid states of shame. As self-protection, they may unrealistically seek or exaggerate situations that enhance the self as brilliant, successful, high in rank, or attractive. They may commit errors in recalling events to augment meanings that promote self-worth.

Characteristics of the patient that might seem hostile, foolish, weak, selfish, inconsiderate, or unattractive may be dislocated from self-conceptualization and instead attributed to another person (Russ et al. 2008). Projection is the relevant defense. Positive ideas, acts, or attributes of the other person are sometimes incorporated into memories as if they were of the self. Such inaccurate portrayal of personal attributes is not delusional (as in psychotic states or mania) but rather a sliding away from the truth to highlight a more positive self-image.

Appraisals that the self is not sufficiently skilled to embark on a plan of action may be totally omitted from a conscious sequence of ideas. This error is, in some patients, an entrenched maladaptive pattern that sets them up for what they fear most: failure and episodes of humiliation, which can lead to self-destructive thoughts. The therapist who tactfully clarifies such patterns must negotiate a minefield, aiming to reduce all-or-none thinking that can lead to suicidal states and carefully avoiding the impression of shaming the patient.

Consideration of the unmet needs of others may also be absent from the patient's descriptions of their social encounters. It follows that such patients often do not recognize the harm they may have done. Instead of repairing problems they have caused, they focus only on their self-advantage (Kealy and Ogrodniczuk 2014). The therapist may use techniques that improve mentalization, showing the patient that such patterns are not truly to their advantage because they lead to loneliness.

Rather than accepting realistic limits, patients may pursue perfection. The narcissistically organized person may have high ambitions but neglect to think through a specific, realistic plan. Instead, they have a fantasy-like demand that with minimal effort they can ascend to glory. The result is an attitude of entitlement, expectation of always getting the best, always being first. This can rupture their relationships with others.

To advance their excessive estimation of self, they will grasp and expand on any perceived talents. Tribute from others is constantly expected, yet the narcissistic person may also markedly devalue peers. Sometimes the ruthless thrust toward self-enhancement is concealed by charm, and lack of concern for others is concealed by pseudo-warmth.

Eventually, the lack of concern will be recognized by an intimate—a spouse, child, roommate, or friend may learn they are unliked or are being used or exploited. As that relationship becomes spoiled, the person with narcissistic personality must befriend a new acquaintance. To avoid that, they may bribe or blackmail the other to stay committed. In that case, it is common for the other to feel restless, knowing that the person's apparent affection or loyalty is only feigned.

As life administers its usual frustrations, a person with narcissistic traits becomes increasingly vulnerable to states of irrationality, anxiety, and depression. Sensing damage to self, they may develop hypochondriasis, depersonalization, or self-destructiveness, as well as feelings of envy, rage, and paranoia; they may make outrageous demands on others.

A talented, smart, wealthy, or exceptionally good-looking person driven by narcissistic personality organization may have enough charisma to take on new relationships as old relationships fracture and perish. They may try to befriend a person in a prestigious and important position to enhance their sense of special privilege. They may also cling to acquaintances who idealize them and discard or depreciate those who are no longer of use in bolstering their self-image.

# Common States of the Patient With Narcissistic Traits

A state of self-righteous rage is common when the patient's self-esteem is threatened (Horowitz 1981; Kohut 1972) and may be suddenly triggered by perceived insults. The rage is a fuel that makes the self feel stronger and avoid possible states of shame.

A well-meant remark by a therapist—such as, "This pattern of demanding control does not work optimally for you; it is like you are shooting yourself down by alienating people in the office rather than cooperating"—may be taken as an insult rather than a useful clarification. The patient may have a sudden shift in state and, in an angry tone, say something like, "Yeah, as if you know anything about business!" The therapist's technique should convey calm containment without counterirritation, protecting the patient from embarrassment and encouraging a working state in which the patient can slowly reconsider the situation.

Another shading of anger may be found in the state of chronic embitterment. In this pattern the person carries a chip on their shoulder and dares other people to knock it off. There may be blustery-outgoing or sullen-withdrawing forms of chronic embitterment. In comparison to indignant rage states, the hostility is subdued. Its source is an internal belief in which the self is being unfairly abused by others or by destiny and fate.

Memories involving probable states of self-righteous rage and chronic embitterment may be fairly evident to the therapist, but it may take time for the patient to recognize shifts into these states. Labeling their states of mind may be helpful, as perceiving a well-described emotion may serve as a warning to be more careful in relationships. We have discussed self-righteous rage and chronic embitterment or rancor; descriptions of other states follow.

The therapist, with time and reappraisal, may help the patient observe a mixed state in which anger is intermingled with shame. The patient is unclear about which emotion in this medley they are feeling, and why. They can learn to clarify, understand, and tolerate self-critical ideas. Relevant concepts include knowing that anticipation of shame develops in response to exposing aspects of the self, such as expressing irrational anger.

A state of exhilaration, characterized by grand ebullience, humorous joking, and charm, is the opposite of self-righteous rage. The patient may feel excitement because of perceived self-elevation through cleverness, sexual prowess, or creativity, mixed with fear that the self-enhancing actions will not meet expectations. This fear may provoke a quality of anxious impatience for praise that mars an otherwise upbeat state.

# The Therapy Process in Patients With Narcissistic Traits

Patients with narcissistic personality traits may initially present with symptoms of anxiety and depression. Later, it becomes apparent they are experiencing major problems with self-righteous rage, the ensuing mixed state of shame/rage/fear, or extreme efforts (such as constantly joking and laughing) to ward off both states.

A problem for the therapist is that such patients tend to misperceive incoming information. Fantasies of past or future self-enhancement are selectively facilitated and overreported in therapy sessions. Reports of outside transactions may be distorted. Although the expectation in psychotherapy is that the patient will be honest, the patient may twist events and reactions to avoid acknowledging a painful reality.

Dissociations may fragment identity (Stolorow and Lachmann 1980). In other words, the patient's inferior views of self are held too far apart from superior views of self, and more importantly, from realistically competent views of self (Rothstein 1984; Wurmser 1981). The person cannot mitigate a specific personal shortcoming by recalling more-positive memories because of the dissociation of experiences. Patients experiencing shame may take an unusually long time to regain positive self-regard. Substances may be misused in an attempt to restore a grandiose self-state. They may bolster their self-esteem by finding reasons to feel superior and denigrate others. Prejudice can make them conclude, "I am the good, heroic, superior one; the others are inferior, bad, dirty, or evil." They may imagine others as "monsters" or worthless.

That extreme label (monster) is generated when the other person or group is targeted with hostility that denies their humanity. An abundance of modern television shows and movies use monster roles, such as vampires, to permit destructive behaviors in heroes (who blow them to pieces with guns or slice them up with swords). We, the audience, have a predictable reaction as critics. If the hero is all good (loves dogs, is nice to old people, smiles at children) and the monster is all bad (kills animals, beats up vulnerable people, rapes children), we are allowed to enjoy the violence in destroying the monster, with applause and cheers.

Viewing others as monsters is a dissociative defense through which the human qualities of a person are forgotten, activating a state organized by a binary good/bad role-schema. This defense allows a person to maintain the illusion that the critic is wholly admiring the hero and utterly loathing the monster. No guilt, fear, or shame over destructive urges need be felt in this state; the anger is an enjoyable energy, a thrill. It is only after transitioning from this state that a patient may become aware of shame or remorse.

The term hero is useful for the role of the self-righteous one, because it also exemplifies the grand sense of entitlement and singularity of one's self-concept when in this state. The hero is strong and feels powerful, and thus the weak schemas of self that have prompted leaden, dull states are more easily dissociated from self-organization.

The hostility in the role-relationship model is pleasurably exciting because the hero expects to receive praise and admiration from the critic for expressing these hostile feelings toward the monster. The hero feels entitled to sadistic gratification over harming the dehumanized other, in addition to exhibitionistic gratification. The grandeur of the self is heightened by the pleasure of merging with the superior status of critic.

These roles are preconscious schemas that act as predictive coding, anticipating how a therapist will respond as the patient tells stories. In the re-narrating and re-schematizing stages of therapy, when defensive distortions have been reduced, the therapist can help make explicit these maladaptive roles and schematic scripts. Mental representation in words that can be logically appraised can lead to forming and recognizing new beliefs about self and others. The practice of new mindfulness and behaviors can lead to revision of unconscious schemas, leading to different predictive coding of expected self-other behaviors.

The roles of a therapeutic alliance can be made explicit and contrasted with momentary projections of role and associated transference feelings. Seeing the monster as evil, bad, brutal, dirty, or ugly allows these traits to be disowned from what otherwise might be a defective self-concept. The attributes are now located in someone else, and the self and the hero are justified in an alliance seen as attacking the bad object. Through externalization of all bad traits and idealization of the hero-therapist, the self can attach and have an idealizing transference. Were the therapist to be perceived as a critic who pitied the monster (others) and despised the violence of the supposed hero (the patient), then the patient could shift from self-righteous rage to shame, withdrawal of alliance, or defensive anger.

A corrective relationship experience for patients with narcissistic traits is one in which therapists offer empathy. They may warmly challenge the patient's observations on what is happening in the alliance in the immediate moments of conversation. The present dialogue of the patient may be angry or withdrawn when the therapist makes a comment that is perceived as blame. A calm comment from the therapist, such as, "blame is in the air," can focus joint attention to the pattern of externalizing blame away from self.

The maladaptive pattern is likely to be repeated. The patient may then observe the therapist repeating the apparent arguments against the pattern. Learning such new patterns of recognizing discord and achieving accord through conversation can be helpful in the present life of the patient. The new patterns may be carried into outside relationships. The patient can learn how to avoid relationship ruptures when *blame is in the air.*

In a challenge to the therapeutic stance of empathetic listening and reacting, patients with narcissistic traits tend to evoke countertransferences in therapists. For example, a patient may accuse a younger therapist of lacking salient life experience. The therapist may feel an urge to be defensive or irritated by the criticism. Instead, they make an amicable remark, such as, "Yes, and we can both learn together by looking at your memories."

When reviewing a problematic pattern as a particular memory to be re-narrated in dialogue, many patients will use intellectualization. In a patient with narcissistic tendencies, intellectualization is not an obstacle. The therapist can use rational dialogue to advance self-reflective capacities, as in the following example.

*Patient:* Well, I apologized to them for my partner's clumsily spilling wine on the tablecloth. She didn't like that. Oh well. [leaves topic]

*Therapist:* That sounds like a familiar pattern. I think it might be helpful to expand on it rather than changing topics.

*Patient:* What do you mean? [in an arrogant and irritated tone]

*Therapist:* May I take us through an expansion, as a kind of intellectual exercise?

*Patient:* [slightly exasperated tone] Sure.

*Therapist:* OK. Here's the intellectual frame: behavior, intention, motivation. Your behavior felt polite to your hosts but rude to your partner, who pouted afterward.

*Patient:* I guess so ...

*Therapist:* Let's look at your behavior to what you intended.

*Patient:* You're so smart; what's your guess?

*Therapist:* Maybe you intended to side with your hosts as "a capable guest" and distance yourself from "the clumsy one."

*Patient:* Yes. It was embarrassing to see that wine stain. So what?

*Therapist:* Now, here is my guess about your not-conscious motives. Perhaps you anticipated the hosts' disdain for you and wanted to prevent a stain on your own self-image.

*Patient:* My partner is clumsy. [proceeds to muse about what the therapist said]

*Therapist:* Mm-hmm.

*Patient:* So I was rude to my partner?

*Therapist:* You wanted to stay in a good mood with your hosts, and you soured it when you put blame on your partner. But I don't think that was your motive. Your motive was to avoid self-blemish, it seems to me. Deep down, you may feel too vulnerable to any kind of criticism when it seems to be pending. When your partner needed your compassion, you pushed her away, and that felt hurtful to her.

*Patient:* Kind of. Can I try and repeat that back?

*Therapist:* Good idea.

*Patient:* If I imagine repeating that moment, I could have let my partner apologize and just nod along myself, not being critical, although I did feel annoyed. But I need not have been rude.

**Table 7.1**  Tactics for patients who distort reality for self-enhancement

| Defensive style | Therapeutic counter |
| --- | --- |
| Focuses on praise and blame issues; is deceitful | Avoid being provoked into either praising or blaming; do not accuse of lying. |
| Avoids or disavows information that deflates self-esteem | Use tactful timing and wording to counteract denials and deceits. |
| Alters meanings about who did what to whom—that is, exaggerates the importance of what the other person did to blame them for what the self minimized to reduce self-criticism | Consistently redefine meanings and encourage realistic appraisals while bolstering against shame. |
| Pays excessive attention to self-enhancement | Cautiously deflate grandiose meanings while empathetically emphasizing realistic skills and capacities. |
| Dislocates bad attributes of self to others | Clarify who is who in terms of acts, intentions, and expectations. |
| Forgives self too easily when some remorse is realistically justified; denies any culpability | Support self-esteem with a genuine interest in the patient while working toward an appropriate sense of responsibility; help plan for realistic acts of remorse without excessive shame. |

The noteworthy moment was when the therapist got to say—and the patient got to hear—that the patient was overly vulnerable to loss of self-esteem. They had compensated in a maladaptive way that, paradoxically, ended up tarnishing their self-esteem. For the patient's preconscious schemas to change, that kind of clarification and interpretation would need many repetitions.

Therapists can improve their technique by recognizing narcissistic transferences in therapy. They range from unrealistically positive feelings, as in idealizing the therapist and feeling idealized by the therapist, to negative ones, such as feeling hypercritical of the therapist or seeing self as being damaged by the therapist's criticism. Even correct clarifications and interpretations can be felt by the patient as damaging criticisms. Tact, repetition, and understanding within a therapeutic alliance may help the patient accept these interventions as well intended and valuable. These approaches and techniques are summarized in Table 7.1 (duplicated from Table 4.5 for ease of reference).

# Summary

By identification with the therapist, the patient with narcissistic tendencies can eventually learn how to be empathetic to others, even in the presence of disputes. Compassion may be retained in arguments. The patient can gradually improve models in their mind of the motives and intentions behind the perceived behaviors of others.

# Key Points

- Labeling and sharing states of mind can help patients increase emotional control and avoid shifts into states that are socially destructive. Entry into a state of self-righteous rage may be suddenly triggered by perceived insult. The rage is a fuel that makes the self feel stronger and avoid possible states of shame.
- Clarifications and interpretations, even when correct, can be felt by the patient as damaging criticisms. Tact, repetition, and understanding within a therapeutic alliance may help the patient accept these interventions as well intended and valuable.
- Intellectualization can be a step toward adaptive change rather than an obstacle to understanding. It can aid in understanding the role-relationship models that preconsciously organize difficult states of mind.

**8**

# Confronting Dilemmas by Assertion of a Therapeutic Alliance

In the preceding chapters, I discussed mechanisms of change used in the therapeutic process. Obstacles were considered, along with ruptures and repairs of the therapeutic alliance. One type of obstacle is modeled by conflict observable in the therapist's mind as a dilemma ("damned if you do and damned if you don't"). The therapist senses a binary of two poles, neither likely to be helpful. Clarifying and then tactfully **confronting**[1] a dilemma provides an opportunity to progress by improving a sense of positive connection.

Dilemmas restrict the therapist's choice of next action. Typically, in a dilemma, the therapist imagines an action to advance the patient's expressions and feelings but anticipates that the imagined action will increase rather than decrease resistance. The technique suggested in this chapter is to self-observe the dilemma and find a middle ground, increasing the safety afforded by instantiating an optimum, present-moment therapeutic alliance. To do so, the therapist explicitly asserts the existing properties of the therapeutic alliance and promotes an

---

[1] Confrontation: A therapist action in which the focus of attention is directed toward a concept that the patient would habitually avoid; this leads toward clarification, interpretation, and insight.

open conversational style on the topic. Some common dilemmas are described in Table 8.1.

For example, a therapist is formulating a potential next statement aimed at calling a patient's attention to an avoidance maneuver. The therapist does not act on the statement because they feel the patient would feel criticized rather than helped.

> Bill has been dealing with a hard topic, his difficult relationship with his older brother, Sid. Bill relates some demands made on him by Sid, ones that he cannot meet. Then he halts mid-phrase, looks away, and frowns with a furrowed brow, glaring eyes, and pursed, drawn-down lips. The therapist wants to comment on the frown as a fact of observation but knows that Bill might experience that as dangerous because he is too embarrassed to explore his rage at Sid. Instead of either extreme of being quiet or commenting on the frown, the therapist chooses a technique of requesting they continue talking on the present topic.

*Bill:* Sid's so demanding! Oh well. [falls silent]

*Therapist:* Hmm, there may be some feelings that just popped up. Has our experience together made it safe enough, I wonder, to tell me more, even though it might be uncomfortable for a bit? [an effort to remind Bill that in the work so far, they had contained negative expression together]

*Bill:* I don't know. Well, Sid crossed me. I guess I lost control, yelled at him too much.

*Therapist:* Huh. I guess you got angry, but you also feel you yelled too much?

*Bill:* Do you think I was justified because he didn't clarify his share?

*Therapist:* That's a hard question, so let's extend it so that the answer is not just yes or no.

*Bill:* [expands on the dispute and his own conflict of how much anger to express at Sid; struggles with his own attitude on what is justified and what might be strategic; feels better about talking over his conflicts with the therapist]

When the therapist recognizes a dilemma in their own mind, they can seek a middle ground between the polarities. Techniques for restoring a working state include making frequent and clear statements about why the therapist is acting in this way. This middle ground between the binaries of the dilemma may be reached if the therapist states the properties of the periodically experienced therapeutic alliance.

---

**Table 8.1** Common dilemmas for a psychotherapist

---

■ The patient is frightened to elaborate on a topic.
  ◪ The therapist attempts to structure the communication of unexpressed ideas and feelings.
  ◪ The patient views this attempt as an invasion or criticism and withdraws even more.

■ The patient manifests a stance of helplessness and dependence on the therapist for guidance.
  ◪ The therapist addresses the dependence or indicates the need to assume more personal responsibility.
  ◪ The patient feels neglected and overwhelmed.

■ The patient is so deflated and demoralized that they have very little impetus to engage in conversation.
  ◪ The therapist encourages the patient to adopt a more positive view of self.
  ◪ The patient perceives the therapist as unempathetic and unrealistically optimistic.

■ The patient feels entitled to more than the therapist can give and so feels neglected and hostile.
  ◪ The therapist is always flexible, makes any appointment times the patient requests, and answers many messages from the patient.
  ◪ The patient feels so special they need not work to change aspects of self.

■ The patient exhibits a tendency to rebel against rules and act out aggressively.
  ◪ The therapist interprets this tendency as maladaptive and needing increased control.
  ◪ The patient views that interpretation as an effort to control them.

■ The patient does little besides repetitively expressing personal suffering.
  ◪ The therapist addresses this pattern and encourages work on possible positive goals.
  ◪ The patient feels so misunderstood that they increase expressions of suffering or even withdraw.

■ The patient is so passive that all initiative is placed with the therapist.
  ◪ The therapist actively focuses attention on problems.
  ◪ The patient complies blandly without exploring meanings.

---

---

**Table 8.1**   Common dilemmas for a psychotherapist (*continued*)

■ The patient is preoccupied with challenging the therapist to show competency and strength.

◰ The therapist addresses this challenge by reassuring the patient about having sufficient expertise.

◳ The patient either obstinately increases the challenge or submits obsequiously and inauthentically.

■ The patient presents in a contrived and inauthentic way in which substitute emotions are used to hide authentic ones.

◰ The therapist confronts the contrived affect.

◳ The patient becomes confused and discouraged.

■ The patient does not express certain ideas and feelings central to core aspects of important topics.

◰ The therapist addresses this avoidance.

◳ The patient experiences the therapist's confrontation as critical and scornful.

---

Part of enabling a patient to elaborate ideas and feelings is helping the patient stabilize their own positive self-regard by seeing an adaptive part of self reflected in the messages of the therapist. The roles and expectations of transactions in an alliance can be repeatedly and simply stated. They clarify the therapist's expectations and may contrast with transference expectations activated in the patient's schema. A generalization of roles and expectations of transactions, as encoded in the therapist's mind, is depicted in Figure 8.1 (a repetition of Figure 6.3).

Once a working state has been restored, a dilemma as experienced in the mind of the therapist can be shared with the patient. The therapist takes ownership of uncertainty (I statements) and does not place it on the patient (you statements).

*Therapist:* Bill, I have a dilemma. I feel a bit unsure of what I should say to you. If I encourage you to tell me more about the bad outcome you felt after that dispute with Sid, then it could feel like I'm being critical of you for not expressing your emotions. But if I don't encourage you to say more about that memory, then I feel as if I am leaving you alone with a puzzling medley of feelings. So I am unsure how to proceed; perhaps you are as well? I think we can clarify this together, slowly, piece by piece.

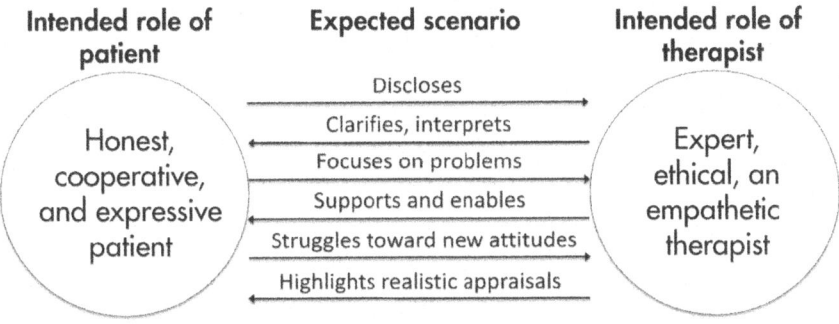

**Figure 8.1** A model of therapeutic alliance.

If the patient does not understand this kind of statement, then the therapist can provide some nonthreatening and hopeful intellectualizations about what therapy is typically like. Stating the expected sequence of transactions may be useful if given in short phrases. These comments might gradually and repeatedly spell out the framework of roles, intentions, and expectations of transactions shown in Figure 8.1.

## Summary

When therapist and patient work in harmony, they can explore meanings, re-narrate memories, and re-schematize preconscious schemas. Observing states of mind leads to formulations of when and why that sense of harmony has been diminished. Self-observation can identify a dilemma in how to proceed in the present moment. If so, a middle ground between the horns of the dilemma is sought. This work builds a memory of the schema of a therapeutic alliance in which the therapist is a noncritical, friendly helper.

## Key Points

- The roles and expectations of transactions in an alliance can be repeatedly and simply stated to the patient. These clarify the therapist's expectations and may contrast with transference expectations activated in the patient's schema.
- Typically, in a dilemma, the therapist imagines a way to advance the patient's expressions and feelings but anticipates that taking

the imagined action will increase rather than decrease resistance. Finding a middle ground between the polarities is the usual technique.

- A therapist takes ownership of uncertainty (I statements) and does not place it on the patient (you statements).

# 9

# Assessing Change During Treatment

When patients ask, "How am I doing?", the therapist often throws the ball back by saying, "How do you think you are doing?" I prefer a different wording: "How do you think *we* are doing?"

While these discussions are the most important ones, as treatment goes forward, it may be helpful to have the patient endorse weekly self-report scales. In organized practices, such repeated measures may include standardized symptom report scales such as the 7-item Generalized Anxiety Disorder (GAD-7), the PTSD Checklist—Civilian version (PCL-C, 17 items), and the 9-item Patient Health Questionnaire (PHQ-9) for depression. In the spirit of sharing optimism with patients, therapists may also (or instead) share with them scales that emphasize positive experiences. Two such scales—Positive States of Mind Scale and Sense of Self-Regard Scale—were developed by the author; readers of this book have permission to copy them for personal and professional use.

If patient scores are low on some of the "good" items of the Positive States of Mind Scale, together the therapist and the patient can establish plans for improving the "low" state to counteract anhedonia. If patient scores are low on the Sense of Self-Regard Scale, the therapist and patient can discuss how to increase a sense of bodily well-being through improved exercise, nutrition, grooming, and dressing.

# Positive States of Mind

The Positive States of Mind Scale (Figure 9.1) is a self-report of the ability to have five types of satisfying and enlivening experiences. It is empirically validated: low scores were found to correlate with dysphoria (Adler et al. 1998; Horowitz et al. 1988). The scale is applicable to the most recent 7-day period. Each item (i.e., not only the total score) can be a focus of attention for goal setting in therapy or longitudinal quantitative analyses.

The fact that the therapist is looking at their patient's scale reports is a technique for giving a valuable "I see you" recognition. They can also remind the patient that low scores can become a useful focus.

*Therapist:* By the way, I noticed on your Positive States of Mind last week that you had trouble with productivity.
*Patient:* OK.
*Therapist:* I just wondered if there are details you might want to add … or not now?
*Patient:* I was blocked in writing an essay on the history of mining. I couldn't put aside my worry about my roommates.
*Therapist:* Maybe we can look together at particular moments of feeling blocked? That way we might come up with plans for getting tasks like that done. We want to explore how this activity can feel rewarding to you rather than frustrating.
*Patient:* I just give up before I get started.
*Therapist:* So you don't make a time to start and later make a time to continue?
*Patient:* Yes, I kind of do. Maybe it is too much of that "giving-up state" we talked about earlier.
*Therapist:* Could be. Let's talk it over from time to time and get that productivity humming a bit more.
*Patient:* Sounds good.

# Sense of Self-Regard Scale

The Sense of Self-Regard Scale (Figure 9.2) was developed to assess self-coherence as sensed by the patient over the last 7 days (Horowitz et al. 1996a). The scores of all five items can be added together. The result provides an approximation of the felt coherence in a subject's current sense of identity. The scale can be repeated weekly or at longer intervals.

Brief self-report scales can be done at intervals. The total scores can be graphed to visualize changes. Looking at trends with the patient can

**Instructions:** Circle a number according to the last 7 days.

| State | Unable to have it | Trouble having it | Limited in having it | Have it well |
|---|---|---|---|---|
| **Focused attention:** Feeling able to work on a task you want or need to do, without many distractions from within yourself. | 0 | 1 | 2 | 3 |
| **Rest:** Able to feel relaxed, without tension. | 0 | 1 | 2 | 3 |
| **Productivity:** Having a feeling of flow and satisfaction while doing something. | 0 | 1 | 2 | 3 |
| **Responsibility:** Feeling that you are doing what you should do to take care of someone else. | 0 | 1 | 2 | 3 |
| **Sharing:** Being able to commune with others in a close way. | 0 | 1 | 2 | 3 |

Scores for individual items can be followed over time.

**Figure 9.1   Positive States of Mind Scale.**

lead to useful conversations about what topics may be next in therapy sessions. Although symptom self-report scales are valuable, deficits on positive scales can be discussed in the context of rationally examining what goals might be established to improve morale and well-being.

Sometimes, events in the patient's life lead to setbacks in positive states of mind and increases in symptoms such as anxiety. Individualized cause-and-effect clarifications and interpretations may be indicated.

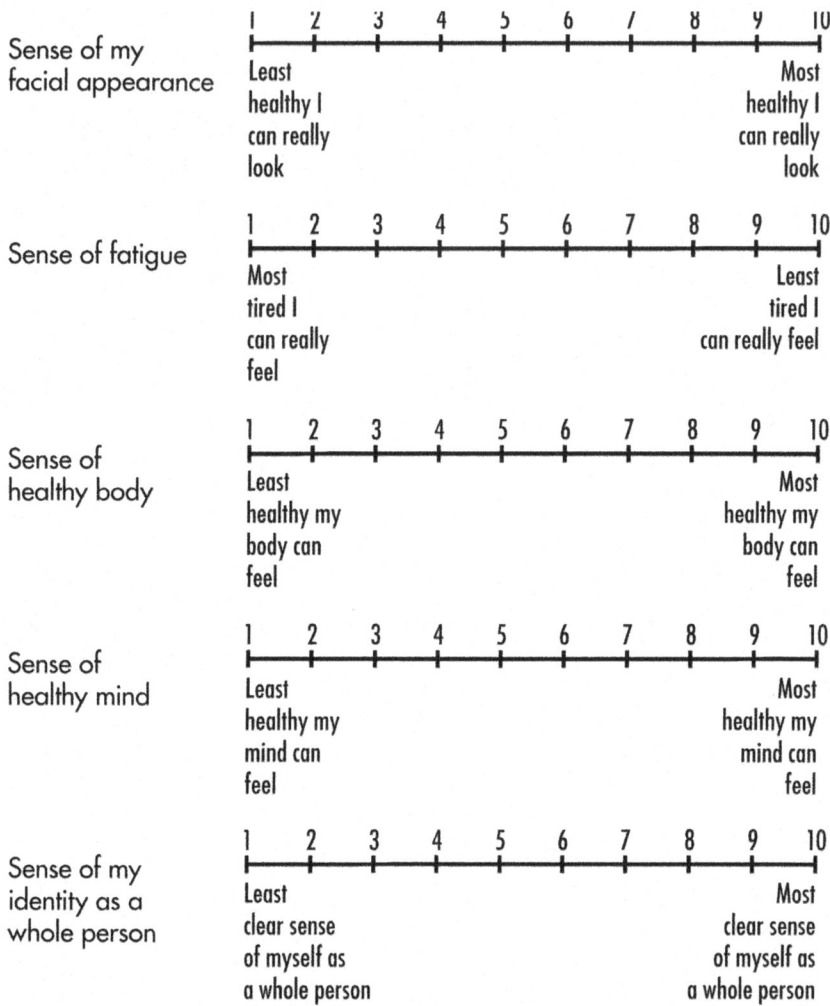

**Figure 9.2   Sense of Self-Regard Scale.**

*Source.* Reprinted with permission from Horowitz M, Sonneborn D, Sugahara C, et al: Self-regard: a new measure. Am J Psychiatry 153(3):382–385, 1996a. Copyright © 1996 American Psychiatric Association. Used with permission. Permitted for clinical use. All other rights restricted.

*Patient:* I am still glad I asked them to move out of my apartment. I don't
    miss the jealousy and arguments.
*Therapist:* You felt you made a realistic choice, I think.

*Patient:* Sure. When I rethink it, I come out in the same place. But I'm not feeling relieved—I don't know what I am feeling. I did that scale on anxious symptoms in the waiting room, and I think I scored higher on tension.

*Therapist:* Maybe you are surprised by the change in your day-by-day feelings since you are now living alone.

*Patient:* That's a good word: surprised! Yes, and what is that? [thinks silently, eyes averted; therapist remains still] Anxious. Not like that social phobia we got past. I fear feeling lonely again. But I am pretty much over that. Just scared a bit. Aimless, no purpose—I expected to get on with work and have found myself procrastinating instead.

*Therapist:* I think although it was reasonable to move on to seek new relationships, you still lost the connections, even though they caused you a lot of trouble and frustration. You asked them to leave. That loss—even though planned—could make you feel anxious. The anxiety may be a reaction to transient changes and will itself be transient, and tolerable.

*Patient:* Makes sense. So, I just endure it?

*Therapist:* Maybe for a time, but based on our work together so far, I expect it will change for the better and your usual courage will come back soon.

*Patient:* Are you trying to make me feel better?

*Therapist:* I'm suggesting a cause for your swerving into more anxious states of mind. From an unsatisfactory domestic life, you have changed to a temporarily empty one. You can expect to get used to being alone and also to seek and find new social connections.

*Patient:* Well, that is a positive way to look at it. Hope so.

Life delivers stressors and losses even to those who have had personality growth during extended psychotherapy. Sometimes, a patient loses a therapist unexpectedly, through death or catastrophe. When this happens, colleagues might consult a professional will. Then a professional may try to help the patient plan how to handle the situation.

*New therapist:* Hello. I am a licensed psychotherapist who has been asked to talk to you by the office of a therapist with whom I believe you were working.

*Patient:* Oh my gosh. What?

*New therapist:* I do not know if you know the bad news of their unavailability.

*Patient:* I heard they died! It's awful! What am I supposed to do next?

*New therapist:* They did leave a professional will asking that someone like me be given the records of their patients. I'd like to offer you an

appointment with me to discuss this event and any further help you
might want. Could we make an appointment quite soon?

*Patient:* I have to think this over.

*New therapist:* Here is my phone number; leave me a message with times to
call you back.

Through therapy, the patient may have more capacity for resilience
in handling bad news, but talking the news over is often a good idea
before deciding what is next.

*Patient:* I feel shocked, but I would like to talk with you. Can we make an
appointment late in the afternoon? I get out of work at 4 P.M.

The example above is not the way anyone wants to end a treatment.
Yet interruptions of treatment also occur when the patient or therapist must move away and telehealth is not feasible. The therapist can
personalize the transition to a new clinician by sharing information
on formulations, techniques, and outcomes. Scale score information
can help the new therapist know the patient's trajectory of change over
time.

Ideally, however, patient and therapist have a planned termination.

# Assessing When to Terminate

In my experience, therapy can be drawn to a close without having per-
fectly achieved goals for change. The closure is one of mutual consent,
ideally discussed over several sessions. Closure means the lapse of reg-
ular human contact with the therapist when regularly scheduled meet-
ings end. Having several sessions before an end point allows the patient
to face with a realistic, adult mind what otherwise might be schematically organized as abandonment. The loss can be faced actively rather
than passively, distinguishing it from a childhood separation that was
experienced passively and helplessly.

# Summary

Therapy progress can be shared with a patient by tracking ups and
downs on self-report scales that recollect the last 7 days (which has
been found to give better recollection than longer time intervals). In
the termination stage of therapy, some symptoms or problems may still

be present. These can be highlighted for further work, on the patient's own or in future treatment.

# Key Points

- Symptom self-report scales can help both patient and therapist track how well adaptive changes in syndromes are occurring.
- The Positive States of Mind Scale can draw attention to what types of rewarding experiences should be planned to counter anhedonia and other negative states of mind.
- Anxious premonitions can be countered with plans for coping with stressor situations, thought through and rehearsed in advance.
- Having several sessions before an end point allows the patient to face a separation event or recent loss with a realistic, adult mind that understands the situation actively rather than passively. This can lead to toleration of an event that might otherwise be schematically organized as abandonment.

# 10

# Endnote

A few final key points may help you in formulating your patient as a self-evolving and self-determining individual. In various chapters, I emphasize the importance of paying attention to enriching the therapeutic relationship in different stages, especially as you convey your empathy and hope. This often means sharing with your patient, at a tactful time, your formulations about their patterns of behavior.

Tactful timing is important in conveying what you have been formulating, because many patients have chronically deflated self-esteem that exacerbates their symptoms. As patients learn that you are listening to them, they feel a sense of increased understanding and encouragement in every session. They think about their relationship with you between sessions and can remember that sense of connection. This may reduce their sense of loneliness and social isolation.

In this book, I state repeatedly that a good therapeutic alliance is a promoter of change, whatever techniques may be used. We regard patients as having individual repertoires of multiple states of mind and preconscious organizers of these recurrent states. Even so, while many people talk of feelings as if they were constant, emotions are labile and can fluctuate. The thoughtful connections between ideas and emotions change across the individual's repertoire of states of mind. It helps patients to recognize this phenomenon.

Combinations of emotions, even opposing feelings, can occur in puzzling combinations. Unpacking parts of the puzzle can be helpful, and the patient can slowly learn new self-reflective capacities. Individualized repertoires of emotions and self-states, however, can be hard for the therapist to conceptualize and the patient to understand. One reason is that for each state of mind, a patient may have different views of self and others.

A format for formulating different schematic structures is presented in several chapters as role-relationship models (RRMs). Attributes of self and other are combined with transactional scripts of interaction patterns that might occur, including potential positive and negative actions of self and expected positive and negative responses of another person. These cognitive structures of self and other may be relevant to clarifying and revising repetitive maladaptive interpersonal patterns, and unpacking these structures can clarify wish-fear-defense configurations.

Formulations of conscious and unconscious factors in the complexity of wish-fear-defense configurations may initially be difficult for a patient to incorporate using their current reflective capacity. Sometimes, constructing a visual representation, such as sketching an RRM, can help increase a patient's understanding. If the formulation is complicated, the therapist may want to share their formulation piece by piece, rather than all at once.

Repetitive maladaptive behavioral patterns are a frequent topic in many therapy sessions. These patterns often include themes of anger, blame, and belittling. A patient's coping skills can be enhanced by helping them pay attention to anticipating relationship ruptures that are likely to occur in the future. Planning strategic responses in advance may reduce the negative ruptures of a connection caused by extreme expressions of anger or sudden declarations of ending a relationship. Planning can help patients develop a sense of the value of constancy, especially in a conflicted relationship that has a shared positive history.

Groups such as families, communities, and cultures may share traumas and losses. Collective grief and animosities related to the group may be a part of the individual's pattern of reactions. Unconscious resentments can emerge as feelings that the clinician may then interpret as belonging not to the individual but to that person's internalized group identity.

Patients may not have had the experience of another person helping them master their anxieties. New skills for emotional regulation during threatening circumstances can develop in the context of the therapeutic alliance.

As mentioned in the Preface, a central feature of this book is the integration of theories and techniques. Being an outstanding therapist involves using theories of change and integrating the theories into your work with each individual patient. Providing effective psychotherapy involves lifelong learning, and lifelong learning is one of the rewards of being a psychotherapist.

# References

Ablon S, Jones E: How expert clinicians' prototypes of an ideal treatment correlate with outcome in psychodynamic and cognitive-behavioral therapy. Psychother Res 8(1):71–83, 1998

Adler NE, Horowitz M, Garcia A, Moyer A: Additional validation of a scale to assess positive states of mind. Psychosom Med 60(1):26–32, 1998 9492235

Aldao A, Nolen-Hoeksema S: Emotional regulation strategies and psychopathology. PsycEXTRA Dataset, 2012

Aldao A, Nolen-Hoeksema S, Schweizer S: Emotion-regulation strategies across psychopathology: a meta-analytic review. Clin Psychol Rev 30(2):217–237, 2010 20015584

American Psychiatric Association: Diagnostic and Statistical Manual of Mental Disorders, 5th Edition. Arlington, VA, American Psychiatric Association, 2013

American Psychiatric Association: Diagnostic and Statistical Manual of Mental Disorders, 5th Edition, Text Revision. Washington, DC, American Psychiatric Association, 2022

Barlow DH, Sauer-Zavala S, Ellard KK: Unified Protocol for Transdiagnostic Treatment of Emotional Disorders: Workbook. Oxford, UK, Oxford University Press, 2017

Bender DS, Morey LC, Skodol AE: Toward a model for assessing level of personality functioning in DSM-5, part I: a review of theory and methods. J Pers Assess 93(4):332–346, 2011 22804672

Bers SA, Besser A, Blatt SJ, Harpaz-Rotem I: An empirical exploration of the dynamics of anorexia nervosa: representations of self, mother, and father. Psychoanal Psychol 30(2):188–209, 2013

Blatman HM: Three analysts on Freud's "Observations on Transference-Love." Panel report. J Am Psychoanal Assoc 63(5):977–990, 2015 26487115

Blatt SJ, Luyten P: A structural-developmental psychodynamic approach to psychopathology: two polarities of experience across the life span. Dev Psychopathol 21(3):793–814, 2009 19583884

Blatt SJ, Auerbach JS, Levy KN: Mental representations in personality development, psychopathology, and the therapeutic process. Rev Gen Psychol 1:351–374, 1997

Bowlby J: Attachment and Loss, Volume 1: Attachment. New York, Basic Books, 1969

Briere J, Elliot DM: Prevalence and psychological sequels of self-reported childhood physical and sexual abuse in a general population sample of men and women. Child Abuse Negl 27(10):1205–1222, 2003 14602100

Brown DP, Elliott DS: Attachment Disturbances in Adults: Treatment for Comprehensive Repair. New York, Norton and Co., 2016

Cabaniss D, Cherry S, Douglas C, et al: Psychodynamic Therapy: A Clinical Manual, 1st Edition. West Sussex, UK, Wiley & Sons, 2011

Cloitre M, Stolbach BC, Herman JL, et al: A developmental approach to complex PTSD: childhood and adult cumulative trauma as predictors of symptom complexity. J Trauma Stress 22(5):399–408, 2009

DeMasi F: The erotic transference: dream or delusion? J Am Psychoanal Assoc 60(6):1199–1220, 2012 23104932

Diamond D, Yeomans FE, Stern BL, Kernberg OF: Treating Pathological Narcissism With Transference-Focused Psychotherapy. New York, Guilford Press, 2022

Diener MJ, Monroe JM: The relationship between adult attachment style and therapeutic alliance in individual psychotherapy: a meta-analytic review. Psychotherapy (Chic) 48(3):237–248, 2011 21604902

Duncan BL: The legacy of Saul Rosenzweig: the profundity of the dodo bird. J Psychother Integration 12(1):32–57, 2002

Eells TD: Handbook of Psychotherapy Case Formulation, 2nd Edition. Edited by Eells TD. New York, Guilford Press, 2007

Fonagy P, Roth A, Higgitt A: Psychodynamic psychotherapies: evidence-based practice and clinical wisdom. Bull Menninger Clin 69(1):1–58, 2005 15899755

Freud S: Observations on transference-love (further recommendations on the technique of psycho-analysis III). Int Z Psychoanal 3(1):1–11, 1915

Gamache D, Laverdière O, Diguer L, et al: The personality organization diagnostic form: development of a revised version. J Nerv Ment Dis 197(5):368–377, 2009 19440111

Greenberg LS: Emotion-Focused Therapy: Theories of Psychotherapy. Washington, DC, American Psychological Association, 2011

Hayes SC, Strosahl KD, Wilson KG: Acceptance and Commitment Therapy: The Process and Practice of Mindful Change. New York, Guilford Press, 2011

Heifets BD, Malenka RC: MDMA as a probe and treatment for social behaviors. Cell 166(2):269–272, 2016

Henderson SW, Martin A: Case formulation and integration of information in child and adolescent mental health, in IACAPAP e-Textbook of Child and Adolescent Mental Health. International Association for Child and Adolescent Psychiatry and Allied Professions. Edited by Rey JM. Geneva, IACAPAP, 2014

Herman J: Trauma and Recovery. New York, Basic Books, 1992

Høglend P, Amlo S, Marble A, et al: Analysis of the patient-therapist relationship in dynamic psychotherapy: an experimental study of transference interpretations. Am J Psychiatry 163(10):1739–1746, 2006 17012684

Horowitz MJ: Self-righteous rage and the attribution of blame. Arch Gen Psychiatry 38(11):1233–1238, 1981 7305603

Horowitz MJ: States of Mind: Configurational Analysis of Individual Personality, 2nd Edition. New York, Plenum Press, 1987

Horowitz MJ: Person Schemas and Maladaptive Interpersonal Patterns. Chicago, University of Chicago Press, 1991

Horowitz MJ: Cognitive psychodynamics: the clinical use of states, person schemas, and defensive control process theories, in Cognitive Science and the Unconscious. Edited by Stein DJ. Washington, DC, American Psychiatric Association Press, 1997, pp 189–205

Horowitz MJ: Understanding Psychotherapy Change: A Practical Guide to Configurational Analysis. Washington, DC, American Psychological Association, 2005

Horowitz MJ: Clinical phenomenology of narcissistic pathology. Psychiatric Ann 39:124–128, 2009

Horowitz MJ: Stress Response Syndromes: PTSD, Grief, Adjustment, and Dissociative Disorders, 5th Edition. New York, Aronson/Rowland, 2011

Horowitz M: Disturbed personality functioning and psychotherapy technique. Psychotherapy (Chic) 50(3):438–442, 2013 24000867

Horowitz MJ: Identity and the New Psychoanalytic Explorations of Self-Organization. New York, Routledge, 2014

Horowitz MJ: Adult Personality Growth in Psychotherapy. Cambridge, UK, Cambridge University Press, 2016a

Horowitz M: Emotional control in psychotherapy discourse. Psychodyn Psychiatry 44(3):385–394, 2016b 27603803

Horowitz M: Redefining identity after trauma or loss. Psychodyn Psychiatry 46(1):135–144, 2018 29480787

Horowitz MJ: Formulation as a Basis for Planning Psychotherapy Treatment, 2nd Edition. Washington, DC, American Psychiatric Association Publishing, 2019

Horowitz MJ: Treatment of Stress Response Syndromes, 2nd Edition. Washington, DC, American Psychiatric Association Publishing, 2021

Horowitz MJ, Möller B: Formulating transference in cognitive and dynamic psychotherapies using role relationship models. J Psychiatr Pract 15(1):25–33, 2009 19182562

Horowitz MJ, Marmar C, Weiss DS, et al: Brief psychotherapy of bereavement reactions: the relationship of process to outcome. Arch Gen Psychiatry 41(5):438–448, 1984 6721669

Horowitz M, Adler N, Kegeles S: A scale for measuring the occurrence of positive states of mind: a preliminary report. Psychosom Med 50(5):477–483, 1988 3186891

Horowitz MJ, Markman HC, Stinson CH, et al: A classification theory of defense, in Repression and Dissociation: Implications for Personality Theory, Psychopathology, and Health. Edited by Singer J. Chicago, University of Chicago Press, 1990

Horowitz M, Stinson C, Fridhandler B, et al: Pathological grief: an intensive case study. Psychiatry 56(4):356–374, 1993 8295974

Horowitz MJ, Milbrath C, Ewert M, et al: Cyclical patterns of states of mind in psychotherapy. Am J Psychiatry 151(12):1767–1770, 1994a 7977883

Horowitz MJ, Milbrath C, Jordan DS, et al: Expressive and defensive behavior during discourse on unresolved topics: a single case study of pathological grief. J Pers 62(4):527–563, 1994b 7861304

Horowitz M, Sonneborn D, Sugahara C, Maercker A: Self-regard: a new measure. Am J Psychiatry 153(3):382–385, 1996a 8610826

Horowitz MJ, Znoj H, Stinson C: Defensive control processes: use of theory in research, formulation, and therapy of stress response syndromes, in Handbook of Coping. Edited by Zeidner M, Endler N. New York, Wiley and Sons, 1996b, pp 532–553

Horowitz MJ, Marmar C, Krupnick J, et al: Personality Styles and Brief Psychotherapy. Northvale, NJ, Jason Aronson, 1997

Kealy D, Ogrodniczuk JS: Pathological narcissism and the obstruction of love. Psychodyn Psychiatry 42(1):101–119, 2014 24555464

Kernberg O: Narcissistic personality disorders. Psychiatric Ann 39:106–110, 2009

Kohut H: Thoughts on narcissism and narcissistic rage. Psychoanal Study Child 27:360–400, 1972

Kohut H: The Restoration of the Self. New York, International Universities Press, 1977

Lieberman AF: Child-Parent Psychotherapy for Preschooler Witnesses of Domestic Violence Program. PsycEXTRA Dataset, 2008

Lindfors O, Knekt P, Heinonen E, Virtala E: Self-concept and quality of object relations as predictors of outcome in short- and long-term psychotherapy. J Affect Disord 152–154:202–211, 2014 24091306

Linehan MM: Skills Training Manual for Treating Borderline Personality Disorder. New York, Guilford Press, 1993

Lingiardi V, McWilliams N (eds): Psychodynamic Diagnostic Manual: PDM-2, 2nd Edition. New York, Guilford Press, 2017

McWilliams N: Psychoanalytic Diagnosis: Understanding Personality Structure in the Clinical Process. New York, Guilford Press, 2011

Mullin AS, Hilsenroth MJ: Relationship between patient pre-treatment object relations functioning and psychodynamic techniques early in treatment. Clin Psychol Psychother 21(2):123–131, 2014 23225502

Nicola SM, Malenka RC: Dopamine depresses excitatory and inhibitory synaptic transmission by distinct mechanisms in the nucleus accumbens. J Neurosci 17(15):5697–5710, 1997 9221769

Norcross JC, Wampold BE: A new therapy for each patient: evidence-based relationships and responsiveness. J Clin Psychol 74(11):1889–1906, 2018 30334258

Piper WE, Azim HFA, Joyce AS, et al: Quality of object relations versus interpersonal functioning as predictors of therapeutic alliance and psychotherapy outcome. J Nerv Ment Dis 179(7):432–438, 1991 1869873

Rothstein A: Fear of humiliation. J Am Psychoanal Assoc 32(1):99–116, 1984 6707437

Russ E, Shedler J, Bradley R, Westen D: Refining the construct of narcissistic personality disorder: diagnostic criteria and subtypes. Am J Psychiatry 165(11):1473–1481, 2008 18708489

Schauer M, Neuner F, Elbert T: Narrative Exposure Therapy, 2nd Edition. Ashland, MA, Hogrefe Publishing, 2011

Shedler J, Westen D: The Shedler-Westen Assessment Procedure (SWAP): making personality diagnosis clinically meaningful. J Pers Assess 89(1):41–55, 2007 17604533

Silberschatz G: Improving the yield of psychotherapy research. Psychother Res 27(1):1–13, 2017 26360343

Skodol AE, Clark LA, Bender DS, et al: Proposed changes in personality and personality disorder assessment and diagnosis for DSM-5, Part I: description and rationale. Personal Disord 2(1):4–22, 2011 22448687

Sloan E, Hall K, Moulding R, et al: Emotion regulation as a transdiagnostic treatment construct across anxiety, depression, substance, eating and borderline personality disorders: a systematic review. Clin Psychol Rev 57:141–163, 2017 28941927

Stolorow RD, Lachmann FM: Psychoanalysis of Developmental Arrests: Theory and Treatment. Madison, CT, International Universities Press, 1980

Stricker G: Psychotherapy Integration. Washington, DC, American Psychological Association, 2010

Vanheule S: Diagnosis in the field of psychotherapy: a plea for an alternative to the DSM-5.x. Psychol Psychother 85(2):128–142, 2012 22903905

Wampold BE: How important are the common factors in psychotherapy? An update. World Psychiatry 14(3):270–277, 2015

Westen D, Shedler J, Bradley B, DeFife JA: An empirically derived taxonomy for personality diagnosis: bridging science and practice in conceptualizing personality. Am J Psychiatry 169(3):273–284, 2012 22193534

Widiger TA: A shaky future for personality disorders. Personal Disord 2(1):54–67, 2011 22448690

World Health Organization: International Statistical Classification of Diseases and Related Health Problems, 11th Revision. Geneva, World Health Organization, 2022

Wurmser L: The Mask of Shame. Baltimore, Johns Hopkins Press, 1981

Young J: Cognitive Therapy for Personality Disorders: A Schema-Focused Approach. Sarasota, FL, Professional Resource Exchange, 1990

# Glossary of Terms

**Assessment:**   A stage of psychotherapy in which complaints, signs, symptoms, problems in living, precipitants, perpetuations, protective resources, and predispositions are considered (and reconsidered).

**Attachment:**   A bond between self and other that is likely to endure. This term is used in formulation to refer to early bonds, perhaps established in the first 18 months of life, that may lead to a template for *secure, insecure/anxious, avoidant*, and *disorganized* schematizations of self with a potentially caring or abusive other.

**Attachment model:**   A preconscious schema of self as connected to significant others (such as parents) in development.

**Belief structure:**   An associational pattern that connects elements of information into a meaningful complex.

**Character:**   Learned, enduring (but only slowly changing) attitudes and cognitive maps that lend continuity over time to a sense of identity and constancy in attachments.

**Clarification:**   A clear verbal statement of a pattern and a chain of events.

**Configuration:**   A set of associatively related beliefs. Harmonious configurations have well-integrated elements. Conflictual configurations have poorly integrated elements, which can be associated with identity disturbances.

**Configurational analysis:**   A system of formulation that describes: (1) phenomena to be explained, (2) states in which the phenomena do and do not occur, (3) themes that lead to state changes and defensive controls that are used to regulate the emotions of these themes, and (4) configurations of self-other attitudes.

**Confrontation:**   A therapist action in which the focus of attention is directed toward a concept that the patient would habitually avoid; this leads toward clarification, interpretation, and insight.

**Corrective relationship experience:**   A new transactional experience that builds trust and safety where distrust and danger have been entrenched as expectations.

**Countertransference:**   The opposite of *transference;* attitudes within a clinician that classically involve reactive feelings elicited by the patient's transference toward the therapist. Commonly, however, clinicians use the term *countertransference* to refer to feelings that the therapist feels toward the patient, regardless of whether those feelings are brought on by the patient's transference.

**Cycle:**   A repeated, sequential pattern.

**Declarative knowledge:**   Beliefs that are consciously represented and can be communicated.

**Displacement:**   Shifting a feeling from one person to another object or person.

**Emotional control:**   Mental activity, often operating unconsciously, that wards off dreaded states such as anxiety, terror, rage, or depression. These regulatory processes use inhibitions and facilitations that can affect both form and content of thought, as well as schemas used to organize thinking, feeling, planning, and acting.

**Exploration of meanings:**   A stage in therapy in which the significance of events to self and loved ones is expanded in terms of implications and expectations for the future.

**Formulation:**   A summary of how a constellation of factors might be the cause of a syndrome that is also being defined by the interactions of these factors. A *case formulation* usually includes the biopsychosocial factors that have led to this particular syndrome in a person. A *personalized formulation* is one that pertains to this particular individual, with a focus on the current interactive factors. A *causal formulation* includes past as well as present factors.

**Identity:**   Awareness of the self as a continuous, and usually coherent, entity that perceives, thinks, feels, decides, and acts. Conscious identity rests on belief structures of one's unconscious self-organization.

**Identity and relationships:**   Schemas of self and others, including attachment models.

**Insight:**   A realization about the cause or effect of a situation or a conscious connection between elements in a pattern.

**Intellectualization:**   A defensive maneuver in which emotions are not represented in talk or thought, although related ideas may be put into words.

**Maladaptive:**   Interfering with an individual's activities of daily living or ability to adapt to and participate in particular circumstances.

**Motive:**   The reason for a decision. There may be motives to *enact* as well as to *restrain* action. There may be motives to think consciously or not to think consciously about a particular topic, memory, or unconscious fantasy. Motives usually refer to enduring themes in self-organization, whereas the word *intention* is used to refer to more transient aims.

**Obstacle:**   An impediment to working through a difficult train of thought.

**Overmodulated:**   A state of mind in which emotion seems to be stifled.

**Parallel processing:**   The simultaneous processing of information in relatively separate channels; for instance, a person appraises a current situation through emotional cognitive processing that is organized by both a competent self-schema and an incompetent self-schema. Parallel processing can yield divergent conclusions.

**Personality:** An individual's enduring and slowly changing configurations of beliefs, preferences, values, traits, and tendencies that make up a unique combination of potential moods, thoughts, and behaviors. Personality consists of the important components of identity and one's relationship patterns, as well as a person's capacity for emotional regulation.

**Phenomenon:** An observable and reportable aspect of mental life, communication, and behavior.

**Plan:** An anticipated way of coping with stress and realizing positive opportunities.

**Preconscious:** Occurring before conscious representation.

**Procedural knowledge:** Know-how that can lead to automatic action sequences without the concomitant declaration of such knowledge in reflective consciousness, operating either preconsciously or unconsciously.

**Projection:** A defensive operation in which an attribute of the self is externalized and regarded as coming from or motivating another person's perceived emotions, words, and actions.

**Projective identification:** A complex form of projection in which actions provoke another person to feel that which is projected, such as anger, thus justifying the self in being angry at the other.

**Psychodynamic configuration:** A constellation of motives defined at the psychological level in terms of wishes, fears, and defensive strategies. A configuration of conflict usually involves a wishfully impulsive aim, a threat that is viewed as a possible consequence of impulsive action toward a desired goal, and a defensive posture that, although compromising the wish, avoids the feared consequences.

**Reaction formation:** The process of defending against one motive by augmenting some other motive or feeling.

**Re-narration:** The process of going back over stories to register a revised, more realistic set of memories.

**Repetitive maladaptive pattern:** A recurrent traitlike repeat of earlier cycles and role-relationship models that, once clarified, can lead to reappraisals and growth, promoting learning in psychotherapy.

**Representation:** An iconic or symbolically encoded meaning that is capable of either conscious awareness or communicative expression. Representations occur in modes such as images, lexical (verbal) propositions, or enactive (somatic) propositions.

**Repression:** A defensive maneuver in which memories and fantasies are unconsciously represented but inhibited from emerging consciously.

**Re-schematization:** The process of altering belief structures by adding new elements, reorganizing existing elements, and altering linkage-strength patterns in the associational connection between elements. The result can modify personality-based attitudes and assumptions.

**Role-relationship model (RRM):**   An inner script or blueprint of interpersonal transactions, as well as attributes of self and others. Some RRMs are *desired*: they depict positive outcomes that a person seeks to achieve. Other RRMs are *dreaded*: they depict negative outcomes that a person seeks to avoid. In addition, some RRMs are *compromises,* used to avoid wish-fear dilemmas. Of these, there are *problematic* compromises, containing symptom-causing elements, and *protective* compromises, containing coping or defensive elements.

**Role reversal:**   The process of shifting roles for self and other to defend against unwanted self-attributions.

**Schema:**   A usually unconscious meaning that can serve as an organizer in the formation of thought. Schemas influence how motives reach awareness and action. Schemas tend to endure, and they change slowly, as the integration of new understandings modifies earlier forms. Small-order schemas can be nested into hierarchies, together acting as larger order or *supraordinate* schemas. Important types of schemas are *person* schemas (self, others, relationship), *event* schemas (marriage, etc.), and *procedural* schemas (how to do something).

**Self-concept:**   The recurrent belief of self-attribution that can be—and at least once, has been—consciously represented.

**Self-organization:**   A person's overall set of available schemas and supraordinate schemas.

**Self-other schema:**   Preconscious coding of the characteristics of each party and the expected transactions between them.

**Self-reflective awareness:**   A state in which self-observation is incorporated into awareness or sensory streams.

**Self-schema:**   One of several potential configurations in cognitive maps that, when activated, can serve as unconscious organizers of many features of the individual into a holistic pattern of thought, mood, and behavior.

**Self-state:**   One of multiple ways in which an individual has learned to experience identity or to have an unreal depersonalization.

**Shimmering state:**   A state that both expresses and stifles—or takes back—expression.

**Social alliance:**   A framework for roles in a dyad that is reciprocal and learned as a context for the degree of sharing of feelings and problems.

**State of mind:**   A combination of conscious and unconscious experiences, with patterns of behavior that last for a period and can be observed by others as having emotional, regulatory, or motivational qualities.

**Support:**   A stage in therapy in which guidance, empathy, and psychoeducation are prominent.

**Therapeutic alliance:**   The relationship that forms between a patient and a therapist, allowing them to work together toward a mutual goal.

**Transference:**   Displacement of ideas, feelings, motives, and actions associated with a previous relationship to a current relationship, to a degree that the belief structure is, at least in part, inappropriate. In the context of a therapy session, when a patient unconsciously projects feelings from past relationships onto the therapist.

**Transference reaction:**   A state in which feelings are expressed that go beyond the frame of a therapeutic alliance.

**Undermodulated:**   A state of mind that is observed to be a lapse in emotional control and contained regulation.

**Well-modulated:**   A state of mind in which regulation by self of degree of expression seems appropriately expressive or contained.

**Working model:**   The currently active schematic organization of beliefs, usually combining perceived information and information from activated, enduring schemas.

# Index